CONTAGIOUS COMPASSION

CONTAGIOUS COMPASSION

Celebrating 100 Years of American Leprosy Missions

Edited by
Edgar Stoesz

Providence House Publishers
PROVIDENCE PUBLISHING CORPORATION
FRANKLIN, TENNESSEE

Printed in the United States of America

10   09   08   07   06   1   2   3   4   5

Library of Congress Control Number: 2005910907

ISBN-13: 978-1-57736-312-5
ISBN-10: 1-57736-312-4

Cover design by Joey McNair

To learn more about American Leprosy Missions or to order *Contagious Compassion*, call 1-800-543-3135. You can also visit the American Leprosy Missions Web site at www.leprosy.org.

PROVIDENCE HOUSE PUBLISHERS
an imprint of
Providence Publishing Corporation
238 Seaboard Lane • Franklin, Tennessee 37067
www.providence-publishing.com
800-321-5692

To the courageous spirit of the uncounted millions who over the centuries
have been and who will yet be afflicted by this dreadful disease;

To the selfless compassion of thousands from every tribe and nation
who have devoted their lives in the service of others;

To the hundreds who over this century have given direction to the work,
passing the torch from one generation to another, refusing to despair
when it appeared to be without hope;

Finally, to the Christ in whose name these many years of service have been
rendered and to whom be honor and glory forever and ever. Amen.

Bringing this book together has been an experience in walking with giants of compassion who gave their lives to serve the forgotten, even the despised. This book is a kind of registry of modern-day heroes, reminiscent of Hebrews 11. By faith they left their homes and careers. By faith they journeyed to distant lands, sometimes burying loved ones there before going on with the work to which they felt called. By faith they ministered to people whose only hope was in another life.

The word *leprosy* is immediately associated with many images, most of them despicable. Among them is *contagion*, driving fear and revulsion into the hearts of onlookers. In the course of the century covered in this book, it is learned that leprosy is not nearly as contagious as long feared. Instead, what proved to be contagious was living among, and serving and loving, people so ostracized by society. Hence the title— *Contagious Compassion*.

We see in these pages an organization called into existence by a heart-wrenching human need. We see it go through growing pains and finally reach maturity. We see a succession of twelve executive officers and 140 directors from all walks of life give direction to the effort. Many served multiple terms, some a lifetime. Those who served faithfully in a staff capacity and those who supported the mission with their prayers and offerings are truly too many to name. They are the unsung heroes of this story.

The theme of how to support a ministry with need and vision always in excess of available resources recurs repeatedly. Many different forms of fundraising were used, none more ingenious than the fabled Pete the Pig (see chapter 2). In the early years auxiliaries were the principal fund-raising vehicles. Then it was direct mail and later, television, but always fundraising was and remains a challenge.

Getting leaders from diverse backgrounds to work together harmoniously on a governing board also had its challenges. Tensions were apparent at points, as there were honest differences over how to address the changing times. This also includes a period of tension with our parent and now once again, our beloved colleague, The Leprosy Mission International (TLMI) London.

If mission is the first word in American Leprosy Missions (ALM) parlance, collaboration is the second. ALM historian Eugene Wilson has identified 182 ALM partners (see appendix B), and he is sure to have missed some! First, there was collaboration with mission organizations representing numerous denominations in the United States, Canada, and Europe.

Early missionaries experienced a dilemma when confronted by persons with leprosy. How could they send them away when even Jesus took time to minister to the "lepers" of his day? Yet caring for begging lepers was not what sending boards had in mind. First TLMI, then ALM became the leprosy specialists, helping missions with this part of their agenda. The first application of this model was in India, but it eventually became universal.

This ALM/mission collaboration was a double win. ALM gained a base for its work. Projects were often financed jointly, expanding the resources available. Especially in the early years, missions often seconded workers to ALM who were already introduced to the culture and who already knew the language.

Missions benefited by being freed to concentrate on the evangelism that was at the heart of their agenda while being associated with a ministry that sought to alleviate a pressing societal problem. More than one mission, ironically, gained local entrée through its association with a leprosy mission. The first Mennonite convert in India had leprosy.

Second, collaborating with fellow leprosy organizations under the umbrella of the International Federation of Anti-Leprosy Associations (ILEP) has also been a boon to ALM. The collaboration expanded coverage and lessened duplication, and it provided a forum for the exchange of ideas and scientific information. Through ILEP, ALM has gained access to the World Health Organization (WHO) and other scientific and professional associations. The Leprosy Mission International (London), ALM parent and frequent project partner, and the Leonard Wood Memorial have been outstanding and vital collaborators.

Finally, ALM has benefited by collaboration with governments. This includes our own United States government and the unique governmental partnership at the U.S. Public Health Service Hospital in Carville, Louisiana, and more recently, grants from USAID providing equipment upgrades at Karigiri, India.

Wilson has listed sixty-two countries in which ALM has worked (see appendix C), resulting in some level of collaboration, some of it significant. Most governments with high leprosy prevalence find their resources overtaxed with a host of health-related issues, now including the HIV/AIDS epidemic. Governments are without question central in the campaign to eradicate leprosy.

Now that the ALM agenda has moved to Leprosy Plus, new partners come into the picture. ALM has worked with Habitat for Humanity International, for example, to provide housing for leprosy-affected families.

Collaboration is always predicated on people. In addition to those already featured in this book, we have selected twenty-two from around the world whom we thought were deserving of special mention, with apologies to others who were truly too numerous to name:

Dr. Rodolfo Bréchet—Angola
Rev. Jorge Macedo—Brazil
Dr. Wayne Meyers*—D.R. Congo
Dr. Luther Fisher*—Ethiopia
Ms. Margaret Fitzherbert—Ethiopia
Dr. Ernest Price—Ethiopia
Dr. Olaf Skinsnes*—Hawaii
Drs. Raj and Mabelle Arole—India
Dr. Jacob Cherian—India
Dr. Robert Cochrane—India
Dr. Ernst Fritschi—India
Dr. C. K. Job—India
Dr. Cornelius Walter—India
Dr. William McColl*—Korea
Dr. Stanley Topple*—Korea
Dr. Roy Pfaltzgraff—Nigeria
Dr. Frank Duerksen—Paraguay and
    Brazil
Ms. Solidad and Mr. Hank Griño—
    Philippines
Ms. Margery Bly—Taiwan
Dr. Richard Keeler*—Trinidad—Tobago
Dr. Glen Brubaker*—Tanzania
Dr. Leo Yoder*—Tanzania

*In addition to major program involvement, these individuals also served on the ALM Board of Directors, some in leadership roles.

This book traces the progress from care to cure. While medical science found cures for many diseases that long plagued humankind, the *M. leprae* bacillus continued to elude scientific advances. All that could be done for victims of leprosy during the first half of this century was to care for them and their families as they waited for death to claim them. Their only hope was in another life.

We see in this account flickers of hope. Chaulmoogra oil made its appearance in the early twentieth century. "Could this be the long prayed-for cure?" caregivers asked optimistically. At first it seemed promising. Patients stood in long lines waiting for shots that were excruciatingly painful, desperate to be freed from the disease that was ruining their lives. Tree plantations were established to ensure a supply of the touted injection. Sadly, the plantations survive even today as testimonials to a false hope.

Hope came next in the form of the drug dapsone. Though immediately effective, the difficulty was in finding the correct dosage to achieve cure without damaging side effects. Once this was resolved, dapsone became the treatment mainstay for a generation, bringing relief to millions. The main disadvantage of dapsone was in the length of treatment required—five to ten years, or even for life. But alas, the hardy *M. leprae* bacillus invented resistance to dapsone.

Finally in the 1980s, scientists working under the direction of the World Health Organization designed a cocktail of three antibiotics (rifampicin, dapsone, and clofazimine). Their objective was twofold: 1) To cure all cases of leprosy, including those resistant to dapsone; and 2) To prevent the emergence of further resistance. The results were dramatic and immediate. A cure had been found. *M. leprae* bacillus had at long last met its match. Not only was the long-awaited, multidrug therapy (MDT) effective, it was available and affordable. ALM joined with an international body of leprosy organizations under the aegis of ILEP, often working closely with host governments, in distributing it to the far corners of the earth.

It was learned simultaneously that leprosy was not as contagious as long believed. The result of these two scientific breakthroughs was that numbers on the world's leprosy registers dropped dramatically. Resident patients were dismissed amid much rejoicing. Whole colonies and asylums erected for a purpose that no longer existed became redundant. Consideration was given to adding leprosy to the list of diseases conquered by modern science.

Alas, amid the euphoria was a qualifier. While MDT was more effective than expected in treating individual patients, its effect on the transmission of leprosy was disappointing. Twenty-five years after the introduction of MDT, the number of new leprosy diagnoses globally has remained fairly constant, at around half a million cases annually. People with leprosy must still be found and treated, which is a daunting challenge, given that leprosy still carries a strong stigma that can be as devastating as the disease itself.

This is compounded because it is still not known exactly how leprosy is transmitted and, thus, how it can be prevented. Only when this part of the puzzle is solved will the ALM vision of freeing the world of leprosy be realized.

Our fondest hope is that this book will both celebrate all that has been accomplished in this century and call attention to the unfinished task stated so boldly in the ALM vision statement— "Christ's servants, freeing the world of leprosy."

*H*ow should a century of service on four continents, spanning a hundred years, involving literally thousands of dedicated workers, many thousands of loyal, widely scattered supporters, and dozens of supporting organizations, be celebrated? the American Leprosy Missions (ALM) board asked itself. We wanted above all else to acknowledge and celebrate God's blessings. We wanted to tell what has been accomplished and at the same time call attention to the still unfinished task. How better to do this than through a celebrative book?

In the process of writing this book, we experienced God's leading and presence that had been so central throughout the organization's one-hundred-year history.

Where would we find the necessary material, particularly from the early years? we asked ourselves. Much of this information was on the verge of being lost permanently through the death of its carriers. Indeed, two of the four pioneers featured in part one of this book died while this book was in process. Yet God led the right people and material to the project. Our hope is that this book will serve as a repository of memories while inspiring a new generation to continue and complete the task.

Felton Ross collaborated with me in setting the stage by describing "In the Beginning (Before 1906)" when the American Mission to Lepers (later American Leprosy Missions) was called into existence. Dr. Ross was ideally suited for this role, having devoted his entire career (spanning almost half of this century) to caring for people with leprosy.

Due to the richness of material and history available, we've organized this book into parts. Part one features key figures representing specific periods and achievements. Each chapter was written by a different contributor, bringing a distinct and unique flavor to each contribution.

The first twenty-year period features the stellar work of James and Laura McKean. In the search for the necessary background material, we learned that Ted Brown had just returned from years of service at what is now known as the McKean Rehabilitation Center in Chiang Mai, Thailand. Daily he walked past the bust of James McKean, determined to become better acquainted with this legendary man. He returned to California, hoping to write the McKean biography but unsure how to find a publisher. Our need became his answer.

Selected to feature for the second twenty-year period were Eugene and Julia Lake Kellersberger in what is now the Democratic Republic of the Congo. We contacted Eugene's daughter, Winifred Kellersberger Vass, retired in Dallas, Texas. She had written her father's biography, *Doctor Not Afraid*. She joined our search for someone to write this chapter and ultimately volunteered to make one last effort to memorialize the father and stepmother she loved and admired.

Having featured Asia and Africa, Presbyterian and Methodist, it now seemed right to turn the focus for the third twenty-year period to the expanding work in South America. The search was further narrowed to the pioneer work of Clara and John Schmidt, who collaborated with communities of Mennonite immigrants recently migrated to Paraguay from Russia. I was already acquainted with that story, having told it in a book, *Garden in the Wilderness,* so I welcomed the opportunity to write this chapter.

Paul and Margaret Brand were chosen to represent the fourth twenty-year period that stands as a crescendo of sorts in this history. Their work began in India but reached significantly into Ethiopia and Carville, Louisiana. When I asked who should be entrusted with the challenge of writing this story, Paul, retired with Margaret in Seattle, Washington, said without hesitation, "Philip Yancey, but he is too busy—don't even ask him." I asked him anyway and, to my delight, he consented.

Part two serves as a news timeline of ALM events and landmarks in its existence.

Part three continues with four contemporary topics. Christopher Doyle and Susan Renault, both ALM staff members, wrote the chapters on Leprosy Plus and rehabilitation, respectively. They helped recruit Dr. Hugh Cross, a British sheepherder turned podiatrist, to write about stigma; and Dr. David Scollard, a well-traveled and highly educated scientist, to write about research. Who better than Dr. Paul Saunderson, ALM's in-house leprologist serving on ILEP committees, to close by peering into the future? Each of these writers is expert in their respective fields. They bring the ALM story to the present.

Part four features the men who have served ALM as executive officers. One is impressed with the skill and resolute dedication represented by these leaders. Their biographies are an abbreviation of this one-hundred-year history.

Sidebars have been used to fill in the gaps. Where sidebars are not signed, they were written by the chapter's author. Helping develop these was Eugene Wilson, recently retired from thirty-nine years on the staff of ALM, which gave him a personal acquaintance with much of the story. He is blessed with an excellent memory and benefited by drawing from the writings of Dr. Oliver Hasselblad.

Also deserving of special mention is Susan Renault, who not only contributed a chapter, but helped with the recruitment of writers and the gathering of pictures.

All writers, I am pleased to say, including the author, served gratis, not wanting to redirect even one dollar contributed for treatment or research.

Efforts were made to reduce the redundancy that is inevitable in a book with multiple writers. We were determined to appropriately recognize the contributions of men and women, although male dominance, particularly prevalent in the earlier history, made that difficult. We regret that it was not possible to adequately recognize the contribution of unnamed and unnumbered national workers.

Finally, we acknowledge the significant role of Providence Publishing Corporation in Franklin, Tennessee, and particularly Nancy Wise who served as editor. She is to be thanked both for her patience and her professional expertise in taking a plethora of ideas and writing styles and shaping them into what we hope you will find to be both an informative and inspirational book.

To all we express our hearty and sincere thanks. *Soli Deo Gloria*. (To God alone be the glory.)

—*Edgar Stoesz*

Acronyms that appear infrequently are defined in the text.

ALERT — All Africa Leprosy and Rehabilitation Training Centre headquartered in Addis Abba, Ethiopia

ALM — American Leprosy Missions headquartered in Greenville, South Carolina

AML — American Mission to Lepers, later, ALM

IDEA — International Association for Integration, Dignity, and Economic Advancement of People Affected by Leprosy

ILEP — International Federation of Anti-Leprosy Associations, headquartered in London, England

MDT — Multidrug Therapy

POD — Prevention of Disability

SLRTC — The Schieffelin Leprosy Research and Training Centre located at Karigiri, India

TLMI — The Leprosy Mission International headquartered in London, England (Also known as The Leprosy Mission and sometimes identified as London)

USPHS — United States Public Health Service

WHO — World Health Organization headquartered in Geneva, Switzerland

"We believe that leprosy can be cured,
can be aborted, can be arrested and made inactive.
One of the best methods is by an agricultural colony,
which combines healthy, wholesome, loving influences with
carefully detailed scientific study and management.
We need to give the loving human touch
that makes life worth living again to these,
the despised and feared in all the earth."

—E. R. Kellersberger, 1939

CONTAGIOUS COMPASSION

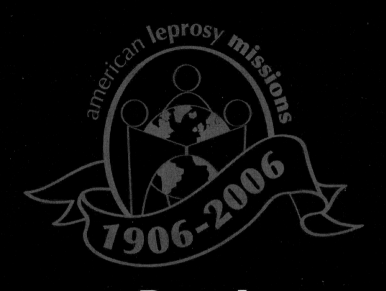

Part I

Chapter 1

In the Beginning (Before 1906)

by Felton Ross and Edgar Stoesz

As Jesus was walking through the countryside, he came upon a man covered with leprosy. When the man saw Jesus, he bowed his face to the ground and begged him saying, "Lord if you choose, you can make me clean." Then Jesus stretched out his hand, touched him, and said, "Be made clean." And immediately the leprosy left him (Luke 5:12–13 NRSV).

It is from biblical passages like this that most Americans are introduced to leprosy, an old disease that still afflicts millions today. However, this book is not about a disease that cripples and disfigures. It is about people—some, victims; others, compassionate caregivers—whose zeal and caring have proven to be more contagious than the disease itself.

Throughout recorded history, leprosy is mentioned. Leprosy was prevalent in Western Europe, particularly Scandinavia, for one thousand years, from the sixth to the sixteenth centuries. Then, with the exception of Norway and parts of Southern Europe including Portugal, Spain, and the Balkan states, it largely disappeared from the European continent. No scientific explanation is available for this welcome occurrence, but speculation attributes it to improvement in the standard of living.

Wherever leprosy made its tragic appearance, however, people mostly looked on helplessly. Eventually asylums were erected, as much to remove these disfigured victims from sight as to care for them. The standard of living in these asylums was subhuman by most standards. Medical treatment was a future hope. Families either hid an infected member from public view, suffering their grief and shame privately, or drove them from their homes to live out their days as vagrants. Life expectancy from onset of the infectious forms of leprosy was mercifully seldom more than ten years.

A Significant But Limited Scientific Breakthrough

The world applauded when, in 1872, science finally caught up with leprosy. Using a primitive microscope, young Norwegian physician Gerhard Armauer Hansen identified leprosy as a living organism. It is now known as *Mycobacterium leprae* or *M. leprae*—the first human disease with a proven bacterial origin. This discovery, though still not a cure, helped to dispel the common misapprehension that leprosy is hereditary. Almost one hundred years elapsed before the next scientific breakthrough occurred.

Gerhard Armauer Hansen

Leprosy in the Bible

The Old and New Testaments contain many references to leprosy, but Bible scholars agree that what the biblical writers and translators referred to as leprosy is not necessarily what is thought of as leprosy today. Before modern-day specialization, a wide range of dermatological conditions were grouped under the term "leprosy."

The Hebrew word for leprosy is *tsarath*, meaning a spot or blemish. The same word is used when a sacrificial animal is rejected because of a blemish. The Greek word is *lepra*, giving the English version of leprosy. This helps to explain the label "unclean" as it applies to victims of leprosy. It contributes to the stigma which some regard as more painful than the disease itself. Associating leprosy with uncleanness or punishment for moral offenses inflicts unnecessary pain.

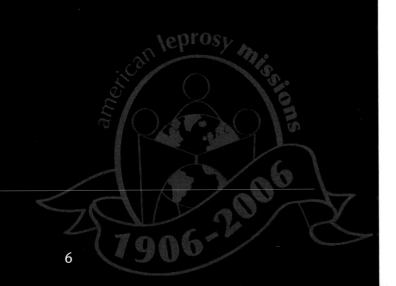

The Great Century of Missions

Introduced by the Catholic church in the sixteenth century, the foreign missionary movement took hold in Protestant circles two centuries later, beginning in the United Kingdom, then spreading throughout Protestant Europe and across the Atlantic to the United States and Canada. Between 1792 and 1824, twelve new missionary societies were organized in the UK. William Carey became the first missionary to set foot on Indian soil in 1793. David Livingston's survey trip in 1841 brought the African continent into world consciousness. The period of 1815 to 1914 was, in the words of mission historian Kenneth Scott Latourette, the "great century of missions."

In the United States, the groundwork for foreign missions was laid by the powerful preaching of acclaimed evangelists such as Jonathan Edwards and Dwight L. Moody. Not to be overlooked were the Wesley brothers, Charles and John. Charles had worked as a missionary in Georgia when he became a Christian in 1736. He said, "I went to America to convert the Indians but who shall convert me?"

Having experienced a spiritual awakening, many felt convicted to share their faith with untold millions who had not come under the spell of the Gospel. So missions followed the tracks of colonialism, sometimes also adopting some of its less savory practices.

As the nineteenth century drew to a close, the compelling mission vision spanned the ocean and found expression first in India, then in other parts of Asia, eventually encircling the globe. The mantra was, "The world for Christ in this generation!" One hundred sixty-two mission boards attended the New York Ecumenical Missionary Conference. In 1910, 4,219 delegates from forty-seven states attended the Men's National Missionary Congress in Chicago. They adopted the following policy statement, revealing something of the tenor of the times.

In view of the Fatherhood of God, the unity of the human race and the sufficiency and finality of the Gospel of Christ; knowing that the field is the world and that this is the only generation we can reach: this first National Missionary Congress in the United States, representing more than twenty million church members, recognizes the immediate proclamation of the Gospel message to be the central and commanding obligation resting upon all Christian Churches and declares its conviction that the church of this generation can and should obey literally the great commandment of our Lord, to preach the Gospel to every creature.

Few hardships or sacrifices were too great for this generation of zealous idealists, driven by a passion for the lost. "The blood of martyrs is the seed of the church" was their battle cry.

Not yet armed with the insights of anthropology, they could not know how their message would be understood and received by very different cultures. Overcoming the cultural screens and linguistic challenges proved to be harder than imagined. Their offer of new life in Christ was received with reservation and sometimes rejected altogether.

Missionaries Encounter Leprosy

While the focus of missionaries and no less the expectation of their supporters was on winning souls, it was often physical needs that captured the attention of pioneer missionaries. And it was in addressing these human needs that they found entrée into foreign cultures. In this process the church community, first in Europe and then in North America, encountered leprosy.

Missionaries organized schools and hospitals, and responded to the human needs with which they were surrounded, including leprosy. Missionaries found themselves strangely drawn to these disfigured creatures regarded by society

William Carey

William Carey, known as the "father of modern missions," encountered leprosy when he arrived in India in 1793. He witnessed a horrible scene and reported it as follows:

> Last week I saw the burning of a leprous man. I got there too late, as he was lifeless when I arrived. I find it is a common experience here. The poor man was well enough to get around by himself. He had dug a pit about ten cubits deep, in which they had made a fire. After all was prepared the poor man rolled himself into it; but when he felt the fire, he prayed to get out but his sister and another relative pressed him down and he was burned to death. What horrible murder.

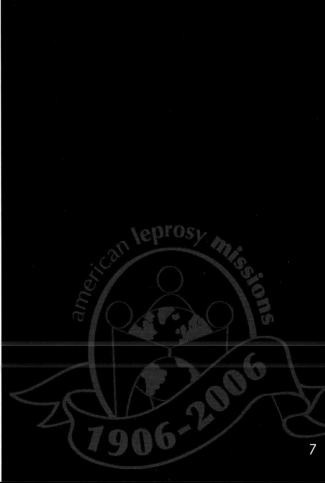

What Are Mycobacteria?

Following the example of Adam, whom God commanded to name all the animals of the earth, scientists continue to name and classify any newly discovered creature—even something as tiny as a germ. Germs are some of the smallest microscopic creatures. The most common germs that cause disease in humans are bacteria, molds (which are fungi), and viruses. In Holland in 1683, Anton van Leeuwenhoek first observed bacteria through small but exquisite microscopes that he made himself as a hobby. About 160 years later, in France, Louis Pasteur began studies that helped scientists identify individual species of bacteria and to recognize that some bacteria cause infection.

In the late nineteenth century, microbiologists in Europe discovered a germ that through the microscope looked like a little rod, but its growth in a test tube resembled a fungus. So, they named it a "mycobacterium," because in Greek, "mykes" means fungus and "bacterion" means little rod. Mycobacteria are extremely small: It would take about four thousand of them laid end-to-end to make a line across the middle of a small coin.

Scientists have now discovered many dozens of species of mycobacteria. Of those that infect humans, the three most important are *Mycobacterium tuberculosis*, which causes tuberculosis, *Mycobacterium leprae*, which causes leprosy, and *Mycobacterium ulcerans*, which causes Buruli ulcer. Even though these diseases are very different from each other, they are all caused by the same family of germs.

—Dr. Wayne Meyers

as "untouchables." Paradoxically, in some cases it was the untouchables who first embraced their offer of salvation in Christ.

Father Damien

Joseph de Veuster, later known as Father Damien, was born in 1840 into a Catholic business family in Flemish Belgium. While in seminary he heard of a new mission in the South Sea that "set his heart on fire." He volunteered to serve with the Fathers of the Sacred Heart but his offer was declined because his studies were incomplete. His brother, however, had recently graduated and was accepted.

When the brother's time of departure arrived, he was taken seriously ill. Father Damien volunteered to use his ticket, but the offer was declined because he lacked the educational qualifications. Father Damien persisted, however, and was granted an exception. At his departure for Hawaii, he prayed that God would grant him twelve years to engage in a mission he could only imagine. Happier than he had ever been, the twenty-three-year-old priest sailed into Honolulu harbor five months later, eager to launch what would become a world-renowned missionary career. His initial assignment utilized his construction skills; everywhere he left behind friends and a newly constructed chapel.

Father Damien was shocked to learn that the government of Hawaii was hunting down and arresting persons suspected of having leprosy and deporting them to Molokai Island with the false hope of stopping the spread of leprosy. Living conditions on Molokai were reported to be so inhumane that it was dubbed the "Living Graveyard." Upon learning that a resident priest was needed, Father Damien volunteered. When the surprised Catholic authorities asked when he was ready to leave, his unanticipated but welcome answer was, "Now."

Arriving on Molokai's rocky shoreline with a small handbag containing all of his earthly possessions, Father Damien was greeted with suspicion by the some eight hundred patients incarcerated there. His first night was spent in the open, under a tree since no other accommodations were available. Appalled by conditions there, Father Damien sought out the neediest. With a hammer in one hand and a rosary in the other, he proceeded to construct modest shelters, including a 12' by 15' log cabin for himself.

"In this place there is no law," he was told. Laws simply did not apply. Sex and drink—these were their only consolation, and the population indulged in both with an understandable lack of inhibition. They were dying anyhow, so why not pass their last few days in blissful oblivion?

Hoping to compensate for the government's neglect, Father Damien faithfully conducted mass every morning, buried the dead, planted gardens and flowers, and spoke about heaven—their only hope. In one of his infrequent letters to family in Belgium he wrote, "I will know I have succeeded when the people sing."

Joseph Dutton

One day Father Damien and others were at the dock to welcome the boat that brought their weekly provisions and the latest victims to add to their rapidly increasing numbers. As it neared the rocky shoreline, they noticed a stranger on board. *Who could that be and what might he want? Visitors rarely come to Molokai.*

Having left the Trappists in Kentucky where he had spent two years searching for a place to do penance for his past, Joseph Dutton was about to set foot on the island that would claim the rest of his life.

A tall man with soldierly appearance, Dutton was clad in faded denims. The night before he had witnessed a scene of horror on the docks reminiscent of experiences in the War between the States that he was hoping to erase. Fifty protesting victims had been prodded aboard ship, others borne on canvas stretchers, ruthlessly herded into crowded, dirty quarters to be transported to their Molokai fate.

St. Francis of Assisi

When St. Francis of Assisi was on a missionary journey, he encountered a beggar with leprosy from whom he turned with revulsion, spurring his horse away. Overwhelmed with guilt he turned back, dismounted, and embraced him. His Christian compassion compelled him to recognize that in spite of horrible, crippling deformity and social alienation, this man was also made in God's image. His missionary vocation took on an additional dimension by forming an order of brothers whose chief concern would be to leprosy sufferers. Because of the influence of St. Francis, awareness was awakened in Italy and elsewhere. Several orders and hospices were founded and admirably served the needs of leprosy patients in many areas of the world.

Dr. Daniel Cornelius Danielssen

Early in the nineteenth century, Dr. Danielssen established a hospital intended primarily for leprosy patients. He was well known for his study of the clinical and pathological characteristics of leprosy. In 1847 he teamed up with Dr. Carl Wilhelm Boeck, a Norwegian dermatologist, to publish their epochal book *On Leprosy (Om Spedalskhed)*. For the first time a truly scientific study defining the signs and symptoms of leprosy was available. Physicians were no longer confused about the differential diagnosis of leprosy.

"Is that Father Damien?" Dutton asked the captain, pretending to appear calm. His eyes were fixed on a man dressed in black, wearing a wide-rimmed hat, standing next to a buggy drawn by a white horse. Not allowing himself to be distracted from his docking procedures, the captain ignored the question. After a brief pause, he offered that Dutton could still change his mind and return with him to Honolulu. "I wouldn't blame you, you know. No one would."

"I've come too far to turn back now." The words sounded resolute enough, but inwardly the forty-three-year-old Dutton was awestruck. Would he be able to adjust to such Spartan surroundings? After all of the patients had left the ship, Dutton turned to the captain who, after shaking his hand, said, "God be with you . . . and if you ever change your mind, I will be back within a week."

"Father?" Dutton called to the man on shore.

"Yes, I am Father Damien. And you?"

"I am Joseph Dutton, I've come from the States to help you."

As they were walking together to the village, Father Damien broke the silence by saying, "But I am unable to pay you." Dutton replied that he would not accept pay if it were offered. Having observed that he came with almost no baggage, Father Damien knew this man had few needs.

So it was that a lifelong mission partnership was formed—two Josephs, de Veuster and Dutton. Day after day, year after year, in all kinds of weather, they built modest houses to replace grass huts. They also built a hospital and two chapels for the growing population.

News of Father Damien's self-sacrificing service eventually spread far and wide, even reaching the Flemish community of his childhood. Wanting to have a part in his work, relatives and friends collected money and sent church bells to sound the call to worship, as bells had done in de Veuster's youth.

Mornings began by celebrating mass, and the days were spent working with his hands or visiting the sick. Evenings ended with Father

Damien singing with the children and telling them stories. The doors to his modest house were seldom closed.

As the years unfolded, the residents of Molokai grew increasingly concerned about Father Damien's health. One evening, it was noticed that he had unknowingly submerged his feet in scalding water without obvious pain. It was then that their growing suspicions were confirmed. Their savior had become the latest victim.

With Dutton's aid, Father Damien continued to work as long as he could. His legendary long days grew shorter, and his resting times longer. Finally Father Damien was confined to his bed, where he received a steady stream of visitors that included many children. In response to his growing international fame, he wrote in his diary, "May all the honor, all the praise they give me, return to God whose servant I am."

Walking became more painful and his eyesight was failing, but Father Damien's spirits were strong. "How good God is," he said to those around him after successors arrived, "to have allowed me to live long enough to enjoy this moment."

On the eve of Palm Sunday 1889, Father Damien received his last communion. Very early the next morning, as the gray shadows of the night began to lift, Father Damien's soul took its flight to his eternal reward. Church bells tolled slowly, sending the sorrowful message across the water and encircling the globe.

King Edward of England had a large cross erected with the inscription: "Greater love hath no man, than that he lay down his life for his friends." It was a fitting eulogy for a remarkable man. His body was buried in Molokai; but King Leopold had it returned to Belgium in 1936.

Father Damien's bust was chosen to represent the state of Hawaii in Statuary Hall, located in the U.S. Congressional building in Washington, D.C.

The First National Leprosy Registry in Norway

In 1849, a clinical research center was built in Lungegaard Hospital in Bergen. It provided additional space for patients, but mainly facilitated study into the nature of leprosy and why it remained a problem of such immensity in parts of Norway. As early as 1832, efforts had been made to take a census of leprosy sufferers in Norway but authorities accepted none until the creation of a National Leprosy Registry in 1856, a historical first.

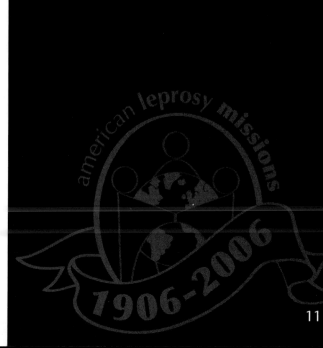

Leprosy Explained

Leprosy, also called Hansen's disease, is an infectious disease caused by a bacterium, *Mycobacterium leprae*, which is closely related to the organism causing tuberculosis. The mechanism of infection is not fully understood, but it is generally thought to be spread by droplets through the upper respiratory tract. Bacteria travel through the air in these droplets and can survive three weeks or longer outside of the human body (on clothing or in dust, for example). The incubation period is generally from two to eight years, but can be as long as twenty years.

Casual contact with someone affected by leprosy does not seem to lead to infection. Most people acquire natural immunity when exposed to the disease, but an estimated 5 percent of the world's population cannot develop immunity. The treatment strategy concentrates on early case-finding and treatment with antibiotics. Left untreated, leprosy can cause grave damage, especially to a patient's skin, nerves, and mucous membranes.

Leprosy is diagnosed by examination, although a laboratory test (a slit skin smear) is also used. Diagnosis is normally based on finding any one of three major signs:

1. one or more hypopigmented, anesthetic skin patches;

2. one or more thickened peripheral nerves; or

3. a positive skin smear.

Most people have almost complete immunity. Others have only moderate immunity that allows the disease to appear, but limits it to a few skin patches. In these people, the number of leprosy bacilli is quite small and they don't show up on the skin smear test. An unfortunate few have such a weak immunity to the leprosy bacillus that it multiplies almost unchecked and freely spreads to almost all parts of the skin and peripheral nerves.

As a bacterial infection, leprosy is effectively treated with antibiotics. Treatment today consists of a successful cocktail of antibiotics, termed multidrug therapy (MDT). If damage has already occurred to the nerves, however, antibiotics will not restore function and other forms of treatment are needed, including physiotherapy.

Nerve involvement starts quite early in a few cases, but in others occurs late in the disease, especially if left untreated. It commonly results in a weakening of various muscles and loss of sensation in hands and feet, so that the person no longer feels hot, cold, or even pain. This leads to accidental damage, ulceration, infection, and eventual destruction of fingers and toes, and the well-known deformities of untreated leprosy. The muscles around the eye may also be affected, resulting in blindness.

Some patients who are cured are, unfortunately, left with residual disabilities, some of which can be addressed through a wide range of interventions including reconstructive surgery and forms of skill training. Patients commonly face long-term problems within their families and communities due to stigma that can be as destructive as the disease itself. Always the goal is to restore the affected person to as normal a life as possible.

Almost every nation has a few individuals with leprosy, including the United States. The heaviest concentrations are found in South Asia, especially India, and in South America and Africa.

—Dr. Paul Saunderson

In his book, *Father Damien*, published in 1890, the British artist E. Clifford gives the following account of conditions in Kalawao four months before Father Damien's death in April 1889:

In the daytime at Molokai one sees the people sitting chatting at their cottage doors, pounding taro root, to make it into their favorite food poi, or galloping on their little ponies—men and women alike astride—between the two villages. And one always receives the ready greeting and the readier smile. These changes have been brought about partly by the increased care of the government itself, and partly by the representations of the noble man who went alone to that plague stricken place when it was the abode of unmitigated terrors . . . I had gone to Molokai expecting to find it scarcely less dreadful than hell itself, and the cheerful people, the lovely landscape, and the comparatively painless life were all surprises.

Wellesley Crosby Bailey

Ministering to "lepers" was obviously not what most sending boards had in mind. Some resisted when their appointed missionaries felt drawn to serve them. This is illustrated by the poignant story of Wellesley Cosby Bailey. Bailey left his home in Ireland to visit his brother, an officer in the British army stationed in India. While there, Bailey felt drawn to missions. He offered himself as a teacher to the American Presbyterian Mission at Ambala, Punjab State. Here the well-known and respected missionary Dr. J. H. Morrison invited him to visit a small leper asylum that he was assisting. Bailey recounted the experience in these words:

To my surprise I found it (the leper asylum) . . . just on the other side of the road from my house, yet perhaps numbers had like myself passed by in utter ignorance that within a stone's throw of the public highway, men and women suffered from the dread disease of leprosy being sheltered and cared for there. The asylum consisted of three rows of huts under some trees. In front of one row the inmates had assembled for worship. They were at all stages of the malady, very terrible to look upon, with sad, woebegone expressions on their faces—a look of utter helplessness. I almost shuddered, yet I was at the time fascinated, and I felt, if ever there was a Christ-like work in this world, it was to go among these poor sufferers and bring to them the consolation of the Gospel.

Bailey, then twenty-three years of age, was put in charge of the asylum. Before long he began to "realize the blessings which such institutions conferred, not only on the victims of leprosy but by removing them from public sight, also by checking spread of the disease through contagion."

After two years, Bailey's fiancée, Alice Grahame, came to visit him from Ireland. They were married and labored side by side until Alice became ill, requiring them to return to Ireland in 1873.

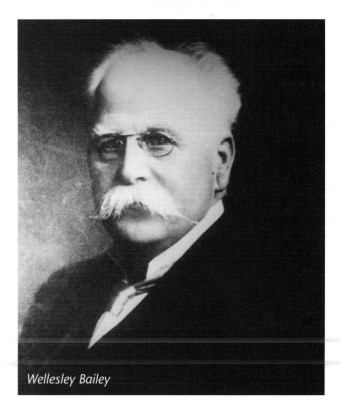

Wellesley Bailey

Language

Someone with leprosy should never be referred to as a leper. Leprosy is a disease, not a proper name. Efforts to combat stigma associated with leprosy have led some to prefer the term Hansen's disease. Both leprosy and Hansen's disease are acceptable, and in common usage, also in this book. We have, however, not edited out the word "leper" when it appeared in the language of the time, even in organizational names like the American Mission to Lepers. AML changed its name for this reason in 1949 to the American Leprosy Missions.

—Eugene Wilson

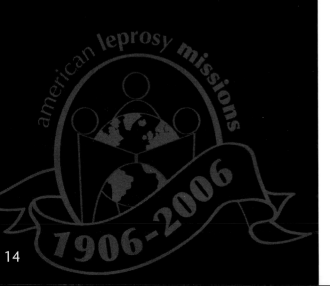

Alice's friends, Charlotte, Isabella, and Jane Pim, invited the Baileys to tell about their work in India. This they did, concentrating on the plight of the lepers. Their simple message was printed in pamphlet form and used by the Pim sisters in fundraising, a challenge they had undertaken. Unbeknown to them the seeds of a new dynamic mission had been planted.

The Baileys returned to India in 1876 under appointment of the Church of Scotland. To no one's surprise, Wellesley Bailey immediately reconnected with leprosy. Not satisfied with what he found, Bailey appealed to the Punjab administrative officer, offering to help with the establishment of an asylum. Without his knowledge, a paradigm had been established which was to serve as a template for leprosy missions— a three-way partnership between missions, governments, and support by friends back home.

Spearheaded by the Pim sisters, friends in Dublin formalized their commitment to the work in India by establishing the Mission to Lepers in India two years later. Charlotte Pim was named honorary secretary.

The Baileys found it necessary to return to Ireland in 1892 for health reasons. While this disrupted their work in India, it permitted them to foster the fledgling support base in the United Kingdom. After the position had been staffed by volunteers for some years, Wellesley Bailey accepted appointment as the first secretary of the mission. His time was divided between strengthening the support base in the UK and visits to India where he participated in opening new centers, following the three-way partnership pioneered in the Punjab. Word spread as calls for help came from China, Japan, and elsewhere, requiring them to add "and the Far East" to their official name in 1893. Five years later, the offices were moved to London where they remain to this day.

The Indian mission to "outcastes" ignored by society found a ready partner in the burgeoning foreign missionary societies in America and the UK. To expand the support base, the Baileys visited Canada and the United States in

1892, and again in 1893. Following the Ireland model, church-based auxiliaries were established, first in Guelph, Ontario, then throughout Canada and the United States. To aid in promoting the work through an energetic but scattered network, Wellesley Bailey began publishing his "occasional papers." This eventually evolved into a quarterly magazine descriptively called *Without the Camp*. Twenty-nine North American auxiliaries raised ten thousand dollars in 1893.

Under God's blessing, the work lurched forward. In India and elsewhere, dedicated and compassionate missionaries from a broad range of mission-minded denominations worked with governments to improve the quality of care. Financial and prayer support was provided by an expanding circle of church friends, often organized into auxiliaries; also from mission minded denominations in Europe and North America. Care was all that could be offered, for there was still no cure.

The Vision Incarnated in a Courageous Woman

Many invested their lives in caring for persons afflicted with leprosy in this era, one of whom was Mary Reed. Born in Ohio in 1855 to parents of Irish descent, Reed taught school for ten years before acting on the call she felt for missionary service in India. Her first term was interrupted with illness. Her treatment and recuperation was in Chandag Heights, nestled in the foothills of the Himalayan Mountains. The natural beauty of her surroundings contrasted sharply with the plight of the some five hundred poverty-laden lepers residing there.

Upon returning to her Ohio home on furlough, Reed began to suspect that she, too, may have fallen prey to this incurable disease. A New York specialist with leprosy experience in Hawaii confirmed her suspicions. Knowing this meant being ostracized, she chose not to burden her family. She made immediate plans to return to India, confiding her illness only to her sister.

The Leprosy Mission International

The Leprosy Mission International (TLMI) grew rapidly and today has councils in twenty-eight countries and a budget of more than eighteen million dollars. The bulk of its work is still in India where three-fourths of the world's leprosy exists. TLMI maintains eighteen Christian leprosy hospitals in India and supports many other projects and programs.

TLMI is truly an international mission that reaches and changes lives all over the world. God has blessed that vision. TLMI's vision continues today to bring hope and new life to people affected by leprosy.

ALM maintains a close working relationship with TLMI. A growing percentage of the ALM annual budget goes to support projects administered by TLMI. There is additionally much exchange and sharing of resources and information. It is entirely appropriate that the ALM's celebration should include special mention of this century-old partnership.

—Susan S. Renault

Recalling the plight of persons affected by leprosy in Chandag Heights, Reed asked to be assigned there. The American Methodist Episcopal Mission agreed to her unusual request and appointed her superintendent of the mission. She wrote her family as follows:

After prayerful consideration, I find it wisest and kindest to tell you, or allow dear brave, kindred hearted Rena, with whom I have entrusted this mystery of God's Providence to tell you what she pledged to keep from you. She will tell you how my Heavenly Father, who is too wise to err, has, in His infinite love and wisdom, chosen, called, and prepared your daughter to teach lessons of patience and endurance and submission, while I shall have the joy of ministering to a class of people who but for the preparation which has been mine for this special work, would have no helper at all; and while I am called apart among these needy creatures, who hunger and thirst for salvation, and for comfort and cheer, He, who Himself, will be to me a sanctuary where I am able to abide, and abide in Him, I shall have a supply of all my needs.

The asylum grew under Mary Reed's visionary and energetic leadership. Not only did she look after the physical needs of the growing community, she resolved disputes and administered a network of schools attended by children whose parents had leprosy. Medical options were few. Mostly she cared for those under her charge and prepared them for eternity. Her census reports recorded both the number in residence and the number of baptized Christians.

No one can know her private struggle, but outwardly she accepted her lot with equanimity and resignation, deeming it to be the will of God. Her philosophy is beautifully stated in one of her favorite hymns:

No chance has brought this ill to me
'Tis God's sweet will, so let it be;

He seeth what I cannot see,
There is a need for each pain,
And He will make it one-day plain
That earthly loss is heavenly gain.

Mary Reed endured her progressing pain uncomplainingly. Hers was, fortunately, the self-healing type of leprosy that left her without physical disabilities. When she was occasionally able to attend missionary gatherings, she quietly took her place at a table alone, not wanting to infect others or make them uncomfortable. She remained at the mountain post until her death in 1943 at the age of eighty-eight.

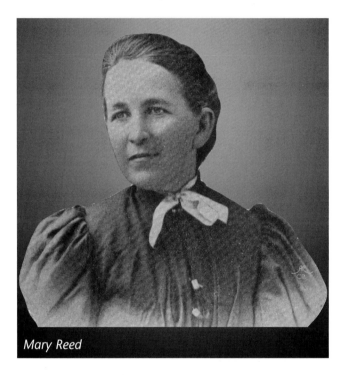
Mary Reed

The Twentieth Century

Church and mission leaders euphorically referred to the twentieth century as the "Christian Century." With fervor and determination, some proclaimed boldly, "Reaching the world for Christ in this generation."

Optimism abounded as the twentieth century burst on the scene. Unimagined scientific, political, and sociological changes were in process. The Industrial Revolution had given rise to burgeoning factories and urbanization. Population pressures in Europe, together with advances in navigational capability and increased demand for raw materials found in the New World, had fueled expansion of colonialism. Though boundary disputes abounded, particularly in Europe, the twentieth century arrived in a time of relative calm, between the Spanish-American War and the First World War.

The United States of America was still emerging. The flag had forty-five stars. Immigrants streamed to its shores by the millions. Henry Ford and the Wright brothers tinkered with what would shortly become the automobile and airplane revolution. Science was ascendant.

Harry S. Truman, Dwight D. Eisenhower, Charles de Gaulle, Nikita Khrushchev, Eleanor Roosevelt, Babe Ruth, Jack Dempsey, and Ernest Hemingway were school-age.

It was still a man's world, but with support from the National Woman Suffrage Association, the Nineteenth Amendment of the U.S. Constitution—giving women the right to vote was working its way through the state legislatures.

Modern medicine was still in its infancy. Clinicians were able to describe and diagnose diseases but the ability to treat diseases and influence their course was still lacking. Such common diseases as bronchitis, tonsillitis, measles, whooping cough, pneumonia, tuberculosis, and malaria were still without a cure. Childbirth remained dangerous for both mothers and infants. Aspirin and barbiturate were about to make their appearance. Antibiotics, insulin, treatment for hypertension, and the ability to control epilepsy first became available in 1912.

Amid all this progress, the treatment of leprosy remained in a primitive state with a cure still beyond reach.

The American Mission to Lepers is Born

The London-based Mission to Lepers in India and the Far East had, under the leadership of Wellesley Bailey, grown to include seventy-two asylums in Burma, Ceylon, China, Japan, Sumatra, and India, caring for and teaching the Good News of Jesus Christ to 7,542 patients and 395 "untainted" children. This included collaboration with American and Canadian missions.

So it was that in 1906 Thomas Bailey, Wellesley's brother, came to New York seeking a stronger support base. He called together seven prominent men in the New York City area who were ministers, mission executives, and businessmen. The historic meeting took place in the home of William Jay Schieffelin. After prayerful consideration, they adopted a charter as follows:

> Whereas the Mission to Lepers in India and the East whose head office is at 28 North Bridge, Edinburgh, Scotland, has deputed Mr. Thomas Bailey to visit this country and form a consultative committee of the Mission for the United States of America, we the undersigned do, at the request of Mr. Bailey, hereby constitute ourselves the Committee for the U.S.A. of the Mission to Lepers in India and the East, with power to add to our number and co-opt new members when necessary, for the purpose of assisting and guiding the Secretary for the U.S.A., who is to be hereafter appointed and advising the Executive of the Mission in matters of policy concerning the promotion of the interests of the Mission in this country, without undertaking any executive authority or financial responsibility.

The American committee held its first meeting on June 11, 1906. John Sinclair was elected chairman; Schieffelin, vice chairman; and Fleming H. Revell, treasurer. A monthly salary of $200 was approved for the services of a secretary. The post, it was explicitly stated, should exclude "any executive authority or financial responsibility." Prophetically, they likened themselves to the biblical mustard seed that, though it is the smallest of seeds, grows to a size where birds nest in its branches.

What a powerful and dedicated collection of men this proved to be. When Sinclair died after only two years with the committee, Schieffelin succeeded him and served for forty-two years. At his side for all but ten of those years was Treasurer Fleming Revell. Together they led the organization through stages of growth, and more than a few achievements and disappointments. Contributions grew slowly but steadily, exceeding fifteen thousand dollars per year for the first time in 1911.

William Mason Danner was invited to become the first full-time secretary in 1911. This required him to be released as sales manager of the Kellogg Food Company, involving a substantial reduction in salary. His children were not surprised that he entertained it. They had observed with others that their father's heart was not in the business world, though a good future awaited him there. When the Kellogg Company agreed to release him, Danner organized a family supper to celebrate the news. Son Mason mounted a chair and, taking the stance of an auctioneer, cried, "Going, going, gone! Sold to the Mission to Lepers."

It was not long before the Danner home in Cambridge, Massachusetts, was turned into an office. The clicking of typewriters was heard coming from what had previously been bedrooms. Although never on the payroll, Mrs. Danner joined in as needed, considering her husband's work to be no less hers. When a major mailing was due, the whole family was enlisted and proceeded in assembly line fashion. The volume of mail soon exceeded the capacity of the family mailbox, resulting in the installation of a bigger one. The seed of an American Mission to Lepers had been planted and dedicated to God for blessing and guidance. It is the fruit of this seed that is the basis of this celebration one hundred years later.

Danner's Twenty-Fifth Year as General Secretary

Letters from more than twenty international notables were received, congratulating the

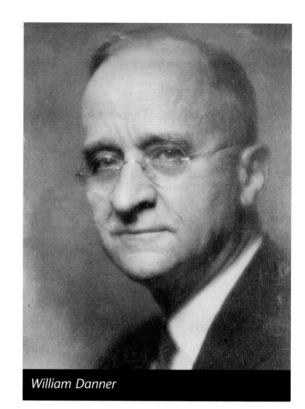

William Danner

American Mission to Lepers on the occasion of Secretary William Danner's twenty-five years as general secretary. Writers included the honorable H. H. Kung, finance minister of China; Mahatma Gandhi of India; Eusebio Ayala, president of Paraguay; Count Kiyoura, president of the Japan Leprosy Prevention Association; the governor general of Khorasan, Persia; four Brazilian leprosy experts; three superintendents of Japanese colonies; the patients in two Japanese colonies; and the secretaries of the British, French, Brazilian, Chinese, and Japanese Missions to Lepers.

The message from Mahatma Gandhi reads as follows:

Dear Friend,

Will you please convey to Dr. W M. Danner, the secretary to the American Mission, my thanks for the humanitarian work that the Mission to Lepers is doing for the suffering humanity?

Yours sincerely,
M/H Gandhi

POST   INDIA

WRITING SPACE

Prof.
Sam Higginbottom Hon. Sett.
Esq,
Leper Asylum.
Naini
E : I : R.

Wardha
15 9/35

Dear Friend,
    I thank you for your letter of the 12 inst. containing the interesting information about the work among lepers by the American Mission. Will you please convey to W.M. Danner, the secretary to the American Mission, my thanks for the humanitarian work that the Mission to Lepers is doing for the suffering humanity?
        Yours sincerely,
        M.K. Gandhi

Postcard from Mahatma Gandhi

John Davis

John Davis grew up in Canada. He came to faith, married, and responded to a call to missionary service. His mission recognized his spiritual and administrative skills, naming him superintendent of the Canadian Baptist Mission in Andra Pradesh, South India, a position he held from 1887 until his retirement in 1904. Under his direction and with support from the Mission to Lepers, an asylum was established in 1900, bringing him into close contact with many patients.

Known for his vision and energy, Davis became a much loved and highly effective mission leader. During his second term, he fell ill and was advised to return to Canada for treatment.

En route, the family, including his wife and three children (three more had remained in Canada), stopped in London for medical consultations. Here a shock awaited them.

A skin specialist gave the dreaded diagnosis, "tubercular leprosy," the term used then to describe the most serious form of leprosy. He was advised, "so long as you do not sleep in the same bed, or drink from the same cup as other people you are not dangerous to anyone."

John Davis knew what this diagnosis meant. He had seen people die of the disease. He knew there was no cure. He knew how leprosy cases were isolated, misunderstood, and mistreated in the homelands. He must have feared that he would infect his own children and wife. With life expectancy in the range of eight to ten years, he accepted the likelihood that he would become increasingly disfigured and disabled. Davis knew he would likely become blind and that his voice might eventually be affected, leaving him able to speak only in whispers.

Davis also knew that many preachers spoke about leprosy as a type of sin; he feared how the stigma would affect his family. Not surprisingly, he wrote, "Had the (physician) told me that I was going to die that night, I would have said, 'The Lord's will be done;' but I was scarcely prepared for this verdict."

After seven months alone in a London hospital, he joined his wife and children in Canada, where he lived in a separate room. He took meals with the family and, within his increasing limitations, helped with the farm work. But he was never again free to express affection for his wife or children with any form of physical contact, although he read Scripture and prayed with them daily.

In 1910 he suffered another severe blow. His devoted wife died after a year of illness, leaving six children, three under the age of fifteen.

One year later, Davis, no longer able to cope, asked to be admitted to the Canadian Government leprosy hospital in New Brunswick, separating him from his family. His illness had progressed to

the point where it was impossible for him to help with the care of his children. His eyesight was failing, yet his spirit remained strong. How was this possible? He summarized it in three points.

1. *At first my disease seemed a cruel cross to bear; but, by His grace and His love, I have either grown stronger or the cross has become lighter; for now I can say with the poet—*

    > *A tent or a cottage, why should I care?*
    > *They are building a palace for me over there!*
    > *Though exiled from home, yet still I can sing;*
    > *All glory to God, I'm a child of the King!*
    > *The child of a King! The child of a King!*
    > *With Jesus my Saviour, I'm the child of a King!*

2. Soon after entering the hospital he wrote:

    The Lord had called away my dear wife, and now He had separated me from my dear children; and yet I can say, "It is the Lord. Let Him do what pleaseth Him." . . . For I was satisfied that "all things work together for good to them that love God." And that He was working for my highest good and His glory. I thought the end might not be far off, and that before the winter was over I might see Him face to face, and "tell the story, saved by grace."

3. A sacred trust; May 31, 1915:

    I have come to regard my sickness as a sacred trust from God. I believe He knew He could trust me with this disease. He knew that He was able to keep me and that I would never deny His name. I have long since given up praying that I may be cured, and have prayed that I may use this disease as a sacred trust from God.

Davis continued in this same grateful spirit to the end of his life. Visitors frequently commented how comforting and inspiring it was to see and hear him, and to realize a little of what the grace of God can do for someone under such circumstances. As he awaited death to claim him, he said, "I can assure you that no bride ever looked forward to her wedding day more than I do to my home-going. I know that it will be the greatest day of my life, and the anticipation of it fills me with inexpressible joy."

John Davis died on April 28, 1916, having lived five years in the leprosy hospital.

P. A. Penner
(Missionary in India, 1900–1941)

Peter and Elizabeth Penner felt called to be the first General Conference Mennonite missionaries to India. The year was 1900, just twenty-five years after their parents pioneered the predominantly Mennonite village of Mountain Lake, Minnesota. With minimal support and scanty instructions, the newly married couple steamed into the Bombay harbor with another missionary couple. As Penner described it in his book, *Twenty-Five Years With God in India,* "Here stood four strangers without a home, without a friend to meet us, and as far as we knew, no friends in all India—strangers, without a word of the language of the country."

"We were never told to work among lepers," Penner said. "Neither did we seek the work. It was given to us by the Lord Jesus Christ. To our shame be it said that for a long time we were so dense, we did not see it."

When the Penners returned from church one Sunday with other believers they were confronted by two persons with leprosy. Penner brought them a plate of food, thinking—hoping—they would leave the premises. In the evening they were still there, lounging under the shade of a tree. When they were still there Monday morning, the young missionary asked them to leave. Plaintively they looked at him and asked, "Where

shall we go?" Penner concluded, "God said plainly, 'Serve them.'"

When the meager mission treasury was soon exhausted, Penner concluded, *Surely this is a hint that the work is not ours!* The next day Penner received a letter from a woman in Bombay with the message, "The spirit leads me to send you Rs 30—for lepers." By 1904 thirty patients were cared for in two huts near Champa, and the work grew year by year.

In 1905 the Penners' infant daughter died. By 1906, sixty-five patients were under the Penners' care, thirty-three of whom had become Christians. Unfortunately, in that same year, Elizabeth Penner died. Their other daughter was sent to live with grandparents in Minnesota, permitting Penner to complete the three years remaining in his term.

The mission motto was "Soup, soap and salvation." What became known as the Bethesda Leper Home was eventually home to over five hundred residents and a bustling Mennonite church. "The results have abundantly testified to the fact that in the caring of lepers we were in God's will," Penner said.

Penner remarried and he and his new wife continued to serve until April 1941, when Penner completed his forty-year career. The Indian government awarded him the prestigious Kaiser-I-Hind medal in a public ceremony.

Fleming H. Revell
(AML treasurer, 1906–1931)

Fleming H. Revell boarded with the renowned evangelist D. L. Moody, his brother-in-law, in Chicago. Moody asked Revell to take charge of publishing one of his periodicals, *Everybody's Paper.* Revell did so, and the following year, founded a company that still exists today.

When his offices were destroyed in the Chicago fire of 1871, Revell reconsidered his priorities, leading him into book publishing. One of his first titles was *Grace and Truth,* a book Moody used for "inquirers." In the meantime, other publishers were printing Moody's sermons without his permission and often with poor quality. This led Moody to name Revell his official publisher in 1880. By the late 1890s, Revell had established himself as the largest publisher of religious books in America, releasing more than three hundred books a year, some on best-seller lists.

Revell married Josephine Barbour in 1872. They had two children, Elizabeth and Fleming Jr., who in 1929 succeeded his father as president of the publishing company which bears his name. Fleming Jr. also succeeded him as treasurer of the AML upon the elder Revell's retirement after twenty-five years of service.

Fleming Revell served on the boards of Wheaton College (1904–1931), Moody Bible Institute, the Presbyterian Church USA Board of Home Missions, Northfield Seminary, the New York YMCA, and the American Mission to Jews.

William Jay Schieffelin

(AML president, 1908–1941)

William Schieffelin was highly respected in business and public service circles that included international and denominational missions. A chemist by profession, he earned PhD. degrees from Columbia University School of Mines (1887) and the University of Munich (1889). He joined his father's drug-manufacturing firm, serving as president until his retirement in 1929. Much of that time, he served as president of the American Mission to Lepers, an office he held from 1908 to 1941.

Schieffelin attended the 1910 World Missionary Conference in Edinburgh, Scotland as a member of the Laymen's Missionary Movement. He was a frequent radio speaker and occasional author. His recreations included sailing, fishing, and riding. In 1891 he married Marie Louisa Shepard and they had nine children.

A Christian man with wide interests and deep sympathies, Schieffelin was an Episcopalian who did not hesitate to take on unpopular causes. As a twenty-four-year-old, he led a successful campaign to prevent New York's Central Park from being broken into parcels and distributed to franchises. He held leadership positions on a variety of boards including the Citizen's Union of New York, the Tuskegee Institute, the Society for the Prevention of Crime, the American Church Society, and Maine Seacoast Mission.

In 1949 William Jay Schieffelin was honored by five organizations on whose boards he had served. The *New York Times* said of him:

> He has made his influence for good felt in dark and distant corners of the world. . . . He has been fighting for good government in New York City for sixty years . . . the interests of working people; the downtrodden and the Negro have . . . been close to his heart. He glories in a tough battle, and has hung many a scalp. We delight to join in a tribute to him.

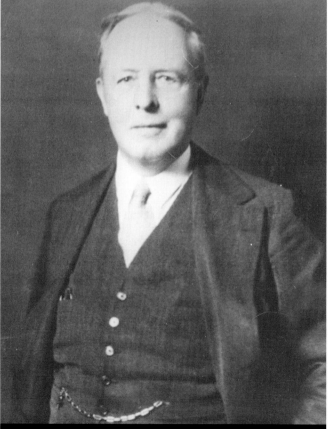

William Jay Schieffelin

ABOUT THE AUTHOR

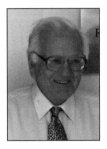

*F*elton Ross grew up in an historic village in Herefordshire, England. While attending the village school, he helped his parents tend a general store. Bible reading and prayer were part of the daily routine. There being no high school in the village, Ross was sent to a boarding school at the age of eleven. He was conscripted by the armed forces after graduating from high school. While in the military he elected to adopt the faith he had been taught and seen practiced at home. Upon being discharged, Ross went to medical school on a military scholarship.

In 1957, Dr. Felton Ross joined the British Colonial Office as a medical officer and was posted to the Oji River leprosy settlement in Eastern Nigeria. There he received training in leprosy from Dr T. Frank Davy and Dr. Arthur S. Garret. In 1960, Ross received a twelve-month World Health Organization (WHO) fellowship for training in surgery of leprosy under Professor Paul W. Brand at Schieffelin Leprosy Rehabilitation Training Centre in Karigiri, India.

Ross served as area superintendent for the national leprosy control program in Eastern Nigeria until 1966. He was then appointed by the ALM to serve as director of training at ALERT (All Africa Leprosy and Rehabilitation Training Centre) in Addis Ababa, Ethiopia. From 1976 until his retirement in January 2000, Ross served as medical advisor with American Leprosy Missions, based at the United States headquarters in Greenville, South Carolina.

Felton and Una Ross have five children and twelve grandchildren.

For Edgar Stoesz's biography, see chapter 4.

Chapter 2

Thailand: Featuring James and Laura McKean (1906–1925)

by Ted R. Brown

The River Ping flows past the city of Chiang Mai in northern Thailand. South of the city, on the east bank of the Ping, there is a diversion in the river. The slice of land demarcated by this river branch is fancifully known as Koh Klang, or "Middle Island." It is the site of McKean Rehabilitation Center, where physically disabled people with and without leprosy are given medical care, physical therapy, occupational therapy, vocational therapy, and spiritual guidance. I lived at Koh Klang for nine years, treating people with leprosy and other diseases, and encountering countless opportunities to be inspired by the grandiose statue at the entrance and to gain a vaguely personal relationship with the man whose image is cast in bronze there.

Dr. James and Laura McKean arrived in Chiang Mai, then a city of twenty thousand persons surrounded by ancient earthen walls, on January 20, 1890. The need for medical work loomed large. There was a void of any organized medical presence in the North. The people treated themselves with herbal decoctions; sought relief with amulets, prayers, and the intercession of spirit doctors and priests; and purchased drugs from itinerant peddlers of Chinese and Ayurevedic medicine. When all these traditional methods failed, they came to the missionaries for a cure. Overwhelmed and unprepared for the throng of patients at its doorstep, Chiang Mai

Mission wrote to the American Presbyterian Board requesting medical professionals. The board sent four doctors between 1872 and 1887.

James McKean was the first person known to concentrate on leprosy patients in Thailand. In addition to overseeing Chiang Mai's first hospital, the McKeans spearheaded a smallpox vaccination program that reached at least two hundred thousand people. Mrs. McKean taught the Gospel to local women and did biblical translations that were later used by epigraphers, linguists, and cultural anthropologists to study the written language of northern Thailand. Together, James and Laura McKean founded at least four churches.

The McKeans sponsored forty-seven leprosy villages across six provinces. The king of Thailand awarded Dr. McKean the Order of the Crown of Siam and the Order of the White Elephant for his work. Ordinary citizens, Christian and Buddhist alike, gave their own honorary titles to the McKeans, referring to them as "benevolent father" and "benevolent mother."

The Making of a Missionary Extraordinaire

James McKean was born on March 10, 1860, in Scotch Grove, Iowa. He was educated at Lenox College in Hopkinton, Iowa. After college McKean studied medicine at Bellevue Hospital Medical College. By the time of his graduation in 1882, Robert Koch and Louis Pasteur had

Missionary Partners

ALM has historically worked closely with foreign missionaries from a wide range of denominations. When early missionaries encountered leprosy in the process of their missionary activity, they frequently turned to ALM as the leprosy specialist and a collaborative effort ensued. These are documented in an unpublished manuscript, "The History of American Leprosy Missions—A Journey of Mercy" by Dr. Oliver W. Hasselblad. One such missionary was Dr. Sam Higgenbottom.

Dr. Sam Higgenbottom—India (1911) Superintendent of the Presbyterian Work at Naini, performed extensive deputation work. He received a personal letter from President William H. Taft dated April 24, 1911 from which the following paragraph is quoted:

> I am happy to bid Godspeed to the Mission to Lepers, which unites America and Great Britain in the fight against this disease, and to commend its work to the charitable and compassionate everywhere.

> **—Edgar Stoesz**

identified the bacterial causes of anthrax and lobar pneumonia, but the germ theory of disease and Lister's principles of aseptic surgical technique had not yet gained acceptance in America. Medical students at Bellevue packed theaters to watch their professors operate barehanded while wearing frock coats.

McKean spent seven years in private practice in Omaha, Nebraska, making calls into the farmlands, often on horseback. It was here that he honed his horsemanship, a skill that served him well in Thailand.

While in Omaha, James McKean suffered the death of his first wife. This loss, together with his missionary heritage, appears to have influenced him to accept an appointment with the American Presbyterian Mission. He married Laura Bell Willson a few weeks before departing for Chiang Mai in Siam. The devotion, faith, and bravery this required of his bride can only be imagined. Together they sailed from San Francisco on September 11, 1889, beginning a remarkable missionary career of more than forty years.

American Missionaries Arrive in the Lanna Realm

When the first Western missionaries arrived in Chiang Mai in the middle of the nineteenth century, Northern Siam/Thailand was a cultural buffer zone between Siam and Burma. The Burmese wielded considerable influence upon Chiang Mai, owing to the legacy of commerce between the North and Burma by means of elephants and pack mules, as well as the burgeoning lumber trade. Chiang Mai mail traveled through Moulmein, Burma, not Bangkok.

In race and language, the Northerners had more in common with the Thai than the Burmese. To their cousins to the south in Siam, they were known as a "warlike race . . . suspicious and unreliable." To the West, they were known as the Lao. They occupied an area of about eighty thousand square miles and numbered between one and three million.

Whereas the Burmese lost what remained of their sovereignty to Britain in the Second Anglo–Burmese War of 1882, the Northern Thai principalities slipped peacefully from the status of *pratet rat*, or dependent states, of Siam into provincial territories of Siam. The *Chaos* (hereditary rulers) of Chiang Mai and other northern principalities signed over much of their authority in treaties of 1874 and 1884. For decades the *Chaos* continued to enjoy great wealth and special privileges, including the right to demand corvée labor from villagers. They were among the most important medical patients and benefactors of the American Presbyterian Mission in Chiang Mai and contributed to the fulfillment of the McKeans's dream of serving people with leprosy.

The Burmese rupee served as the currency, not the Siamese tical or bath, prompting one traveler to comment, "No Siamese coin is ever seen there, and it would not be accepted if tendered." The royal family of Chiang Mai was as likely to send its sons to Burma to be educated as to Bangkok.

The earliest missionaries to Northern Thailand were Buddhists from India or Sri Lanka. The first Christian missionaries to visit Chiang Mai were the French Catholic priests M. Grandjean and M. Vachal. Arriving in January 1844, they were not immediately encouraged by the prospects. Throughout their journey, they met with hardship and deprivation. When they returned to Bangkok later that year, Grandjean found that his hair had grayed and he had aged such that he was referred to as "Old Father."

Reverend Daniel and Mrs. Sophia McGilvary were the first Protestant missionaries to Chiang Mai, arriving in 1858. Daniel McGilvary was a North Carolinian who had studied at Princeton Seminary before dedicating his life to missionary work. In Bangkok, he met his bride, Sophia Royce Bradley, the eldest daughter of the preeminent Dr. Bradley, another early-American missionary. After years of proselytizing in Petchburi, the McGilvarys and their two children bravely set out for Chiang Mai, reaching the city by riverboat on April 3, 1867. Staying at an open rest house, they began preaching the Gospel and sowing the seeds of faith. Having grown up in Thailand, Sophia was of great help to her husband in learning the Northern dialect; interacting with the curious villagers who were constantly observing the strange white people; and in sustaining a family with food and items of daily living found locally. Years later, the McKeans arrived to carry on the McGilvarys' work.

The Challenge of Leprosy

"Neither history nor legend hint as to the time and manner in which leprosy came into Siam," wrote James McKean. It is probable that the disease came with the Thai people as they moved downwards from China over several centuries. There are no records of the presence or absence of leprosy in southern China through the T'ang Dynasty (619-907 C.E.), but that still leaves ample centuries to satisfy McKean's theory. A Chinese name for leprosy is "Great Wind Disease." This is the exact meaning of an old name for leprosy used in northern Thailand: *lom luang*, giving further etymological credence to McKean's view.

Until taught otherwise by public health campaigners, Thais assumed that leprosy was hereditary or due to the wrath of spirits. Without conceiving leprosy as a public health menace, ordinary people saw no threat in the disease. That is not to say people did not find other reasons to ostracize leprosy sufferers. In the traditional society of northern Thailand, leprosy victims were called *chow khi toot*, roughly translatable as "filthy lepers." They may have been more ostracized in the northern than in the southern or central regions of Siam. I have spoken with many people there who contracted leprosy in their youth. One man commented having felt almost subhuman when he was taunted with, "Here comes the filthy leper."

In the McKeans's time, persons with leprosy could expect little kindness. They were regarded

Childhood of Leprosy

One leprosy patient, Elder Yui Thepniran, wrote of his childhood in the 1920s as follows:

It was unbearable both in mind and body since I had no real home, or proper food, even though I was at this tender age (eleven). During the daytime I hid in the jungle far away from the village. At night, alone, fearing wild animals (Nan was tiger territory) and other terrors of the dark, I would slip back home unseen by the neighbors. Even so, my neighbors were pitiless. They treated both my father and me badly, spitting in our faces, stoning our house, and damaging our crops. They even killed our animals. Such was my early life spent amongst that ignorant and superstitious people.

as walking corpses. In McKean's words, they were "hated and feared, tragic figures dragging their weary bodies from place to place." Once the disease was advanced, they became unable to work. The stigma of leprosy made life within the village impossible and fractured what family and social supports they had.

McKean, the most knowledgeable leprosy expert of his day in Thailand, thought the disease was not hereditary, that it was infectious only to some individuals while the rest were immune to the disease, and that it was transmitted only by "prolonged and intimate contact."

In the early 1900s, leprosy was viewed as an insidious disease that was practically always fatal. Estimates of world leprosy prevalence between 1900 and 1928 were two to three million. When Thailand made its first census in 1909, the Leprosy Division estimated ten thousand cases of leprosy for the entire country. Two years later, McKean raised that estimate to fifteen thousand, and in 1930, to twenty thousand cases. With the Thai population at ten to eleven million, that computes to a prevalence of one in five hundred.

In 1921 the northern Thailand province of Payap Circle, which included Chiang Mai, Chiang Rai, Lamphun, and Mae Hong Son, had 831 registered cases. There were high concentrations in some northern areas, particularly Nan Province. In 1914, Dr. S. C. Peoples stated it was "pretty well filled up with them (leprosy cases): the condition is terrible." Rev. Hugh Taylor noted, "I found the district (Muang Yome, Nan Province) full of lepers. I would not dare make a guess how many hundreds there were." He wrote of a village where over half of the households had someone with leprosy.

McKean, an orphan himself, took the plight of those with leprosy personally. He wrote, "On more than one occasion I found these poor outcasts lying dead in the public rest houses where they had gone for the night. Their need touched me greatly. No helping hand was stretched out to them." Within a year or two of the McKeans's arrival, the Chiang Mai missionaries began helping the "wandering lepers" with weekly distributions of pennies and medicine, and offered handouts of clothing during the cold season. McKean made no boasts about the relief, which he described as "desultory and ineffective aid." He once told a young missionary that he began his leprosy work with two dollars and that might well have been true.

People with leprosy came to regard McKean as their patron. He wrote, "Finding that their requests met with response, they came in increasing numbers and in increasing frequency so that during a period of several years not a day passed in which leper beggars, in companies of from two to a dozen or more persons, did not come for alms." Those who sought leprosy care at the American Hospital were not turned away, but were carried out into the road to have their wounds dressed or provided with temporary rooms outside of the hospital wards. Simply allowing them to beg in front of the American Hospital without shooing them away was an act of charity.

The Need Called For Response

By 1903, 50 to 150 leprosy victims had established an encampment on an island in the Ping River one mile south of Chiang Mai. When someone was discovered to have leprosy, they were banished to the island, where McKean ministered to their needs. The Chiang Mai church occasionally provided sustenance, clothing, and Christian books. However, in 1905, under unknown circumstances, the people were driven from the island and left homeless.

With the number of persons with leprosy presenting themselves for care increasing annually, McKean felt a pressing need to find a permanent home for society's outcasts. The answer to his prayers sprang from the very peculiar circumstances surrounding a rogue elephant.

Elephants have held a lofty status throughout Thai history. The flag of the kingdom of Siam includes an image of an elephant, and elephants were auspicious and felicitous gifts. The events leading to the collapse of Ayutthaya, the ancient capital of Siam, began with a refusal to send four white elephants to Burma as a token of homage. King Mongkut, who was King Rama IV, once offered to send President Lincoln a herd of elephants for breeding purposes to solve America's transportation problem.

James McKean

So it was that a very unruly elephant opened the door to better care for people afflicted with leprosy. This elephant had become uncontrollable and killed several of its keepers. Being a royal elephant, however, it could not be destroyed. His front legs were hobbled with a heavy chain and he was imprisoned on Koh Klang, the "middle island" on the east bank of the Ping River. There he showed not the slightest respect for his human neighbors. When he wanted rice, he tore down the granary. If a house stood in his way, he pushed it over and went on. The people abandoned the island out of fear, leaving the elephant as its sole occupant for the next thirty years. Even after its death in 1905, people were afraid to reinhabit the island for fear of the elephant's ghost, leaving the island an overgrown wilderness.

Chantah Indravude, assistant to Rev. Daniel McGilvary when the McKeans first came to Thailand, had suggested that Koh Klang might be used as a leprosy asylum. Chantah had seen

An Island for a Pair of Red Slippers

There is a fable that Dr. McKean was visiting the prince of Chiang Mai while wearing red slippers. Guests were expected to doff their shoes when in the palace and McKean may have brought the slippers to fit the occasion. When the prince complimented his fine footwear, Dr. McKean made a gift of the slippers. In return, the prince granted his wish to make a home for those with leprosy. Lutz Hartdegan, who put this myth in print added, "The red velvet slippers had cost the old man two dollars—that was the price of the island."

the island and learned its story while making a river voyage. In late 1905, McKean, now forty-seven years of age, had an audience in Bangkok with H.R.H. Prince Damrong, who was the minister of the interior of Siam. He presented his plan for Koh Klang. In succession, Prince Damrong, then next the high commissioner of Chiang Mai, and finally, the prince of Chiang Mai himself agreed to McKean's proposal. Thus, Thailand's first leprosy center was birthed in the same year the American Mission to Lepers was founded.

There are two versions of what *Chao* (Prince) Inthawarorot Suriyawong said to McKean when he gave formal permission. One source records the prince's words as, "Very well then. Now, Nakorn Ping [Chiang Mai] will be a cleaner place, too." Another description is more poignant, but perhaps also apocryphal. It goes: "Why, Dr. McKean, are you going to take care of those who are already dead?" McKean did not record the exact words of the prince, the former owner of the mad elephant of Koh Klang. McKean simply remarked that the prince was "generous in a marked degree."

Lepers Obtain a Refuge

The Presbyterian Mission was granted 400 rai (164 acres) on the southern half of Koh Klang Island. Developing it into a village for leprosy sufferers was not a simple process because the land rights were unclear. By tradition, the ruler of Chiang Mai owned the forests of all property in the area. He could therefore sell the timber rights to whomever he pleased.

The people of the immediate neighborhood were not thrilled to have a leprosy asylum in their midst. They secretly broke a dam one night that temporarily flooded the island. Again, difficulties were smoothed out, this time with help from the Siamese commissioner, Chao Phraya Surasi Wisitsak.

Announcing the exciting news to supporters in the U.S., McKean wrote, "Surely the time is ripe for the beginning of a Leper Refuge in Siam. We have the land; we have the lepers in abundance." A call was made for donations. In October 1907, McKean and Chantah Indravude floated on a bamboo raft along the Ping River to explore their would-be asylum. They wanted to put ashore at the north end of Koh Klang, but the pole man refused, saying that a wicked, fierce elephant inhabited the area. (He must not have known that it had already died.) They went to the location that one day would become Cottage #14 of South Village One, and there they knelt and prayed.

Laborers from the local Bah Kluei village were hired and spent several months making a clearing and building bamboo huts with thatched roofs. In 1908, McKean and Chantah went into the city and invited the leprosy victims who were begging along the Ping River and sleeping under a bridge to live at Koh Klong. They promised to bring rice, dry food, salt, dried meat, and roasted fish once a week and to also provide them with medications. Money was used to persuade some individuals and families to come.

Seven leprosy victims and two children moved to the island. Not much knowledge of this small band of homesteaders has been preserved. One of them had appeared at the American Hospital with a gangrenous foot requiring amputation. A second colonizer died within weeks. A third, Khun Kaeo (the only woman and the only one whose name has been preserved) was already a Christian. Her husband, who was badly deformed and disabled, joined her on the island.

Leprosy Care Finally Integrated into the Mission

During 1909 the population increased from eight to fifteen, despite two deaths. By 1910, its number had grown to twenty. For several years, the community had no road access. New arrivals had to come by boat. Nevertheless, the population continued to grow rapidly. Parenthetically, McKean wrote that the new arrivals were not professional beggars, whose way of living would only be altered by the threat of imprisonment. Instead, they were mostly people who had been hidden away by their families, living in unseen internal exile within homes and villages throughout the North.

In February 1909, the McKeans went to New York to attend to Mrs. McKean's failing health. Before returning the next year, McKean spent two months studying tropical disease in England. Another fortnight was spent visiting hospitals and leprosy asylums in India and Burma. He returned with new ideas of how to organize a leprosarium and with thirteen thousand dollars in donations.

During McKean's absence, Chantah wooed a wealthy Burmese resident of Chiang Mai to raise funds for two permanent dormitories. He also hired Loong Paeng and his wife as non-leprosy caretakers and Christian leaders. Two of Loong Paeng's children had leprosy and were among the first residents, so he was naturally sympathetic. Loong Paeng remained as caretaker until his death in 1915.

When McKean returned, voices within the Presbyterian Mission still considered the asylum an "extra-mission institution" and wanted to have little to do with it. Persisting, McKean received permission to build the first permanent structures. They were cement and brick buildings, one for male and one for female patients. McKean's architectural designs, it was said, were based on what he saw in India.

The difficult work of clearing the dense overgrowth and leveling the plain was undertaken without the aid of a bulldozer; laborers from the surrounding areas were hired to tackle this problem with shovels and hoes. The standard construction materials were wood and bamboo since superstition mitigated against building with bricks, except for monasteries and temples. There were no merchants from whom bricks could be locally bought.

This obstacle was overcome when an American brick-making machine, designed by Henry Martin of Lancaster, Pennsylvania, was discovered. It made bricks out of clay and was powered not by steam, but by slow-moving water buffalos. Brick making eventually became one of the commercial industries at the leprosy asylum. By 1930, the asylum was producing three hundred thousand bricks annually.

By the beginning of 1914, four more buildings had been added, each with sixteen-bed capacity and reserved for disabled invalids. A bamboo chapel had been in place since the first year.

Chiang Mai Leper Asylum

With more than one thousand persons in attendance, the asylum was opened on June 11, 1913. The ceremony included high government officials for the North and Chao Kaeo Nawarat, the ninth prince of the Kawila dynasty. Leprosy patients numbering 139 had been admitted, of which 100 remained.

A sign over the asylum read in Thai, "Koh Klang Hospital." It was thought of as both a hospital and a colony for leprosy, the only place of its kind in the North. Distinct from the many leprosy villages scattered around the North, it was not hidden. Most everyone in the North had heard of it and knew its function. Koh Klang was consequently subject to derision. Conversely, being well known, the leprosarium attracted victims from far and wide.

Full of trepidation, patients came seeking refuge more often than treatment. McKean observed, "So long as one is allowed to live in his own home he will not seek the asylum. It is only when his presence becomes unendurable and when family love has been extinguished by the loathsomeness of the disease that the miserable person comes to us."

The truth about the Chiang Mai Leper Asylum was brighter than public perceptions. It was not a house of horrors where people were quarantined. It was instead a unique commune. The society was not self-sustaining like a kibbutz, because there was little organized, profitable industry. Support from the Presbyterian Mission, the American Mission to Lepers, and foreign benefactors, plus an annual stipend of 9,000 baht from the Thai government provided a continual infusion of funds to sustain the community.

The inhabitants received a weekly allowance, then equivalent to 40 cents, sufficient to buy their weekly food. It exceeded what they could expect in their village. They were given shelter, clothing, and—most important—social acceptance and love. One grateful resident recalled the words spoken to her when admitted to the clinic as a thirteen-year-old, "You can stay here now and study and then work in a peaceful place." Another resident explained they had been ostracized by their home communities and in most cases, rejected by their family as well. Who would want to live under those circumstances? Most who came to their new home accepted Christianity as their faith. This, in a Buddhist setting, served to unite them.

The community lived then (as it does today) under a set of rules and moral requirements, some of which were imposed due to fear of contagion and others according to Christian ideals. There were rules about how their houses and gardens should be maintained and about where to hang the laundry to keep the villages looking neat and orderly. There was an ever-present pass system and a 10:00 P.M. curfew. Gambling, drinking alcohol, and fighting were strictly forbidden.

Stick-toting guards were employed to enforce these rules. If a man was caught sneaking into the women's village, the case was reported to the headman, who consulted the director. Such an offense might require carrying one-third of a wagonload of sand out of the Ping River to the sand pile. The guilty party's sweetheart might help to carry the load.

In the early years, leprosy residents were regarded as guests. Paid non-leprosy employees moved into the neighborhood and did much of the work. Gradually, McKean determined to turn the work of the asylum over to the patients themselves. Putting the inhabitants to work was seen as occupational therapy in the truest sense of the word. "In selected cases," McKean said, "the provisions of the Asylum which afford good food, good cheer, physical comfort, freedom of worry and a proper amount of physical labor are of paramount value in bringing about an arrested or negative phase of the disease; and that in such cases specific medication possibly is of minor value." In weighing this statement, bear in mind that at the time of its writing no cures were possible.

Support was initially from local Thai and foreign donors living in the area. The first overseas support was received in 1909 when £120 was received from the Mission to the Lepers in India and the East, later known as the Leprosy Mission, based in London. It remained the main foreign supporter until 1917 when this role was assumed by what became known as the American Leprosy Missions. These two organizations provided most of the funding for buildings and maintenance. In 1919 the Thai government contributed 10,000 baht, which became an annual gift throughout the 1920s and 1930s.

One of the first dormitories was designated as an infirmary. There was little to distinguish this building other than white crosses decorating the frieze and the presence of nurse aides, both male and female. Treatment was limited to wound care. McKean was overworked at the time by other evangelical and medical obligations, causing his health to deteriorate. He left on furlough in July 1915 and did not return until late 1917, when he was found to have tuberculosis, a common condition among the American missionaries at the time.

A Cure, At Last?

During McKean's absence, the first attempts to treat leprosy were initiated by the acting mission superintendent, Dr. E. C. Cort. Experimentation with chaulmoogra oil injections was offered "to all who care for it." Nine men volunteered. The right doses were worked out by trial and error since the medication could induce severe reactions. The medicine was brought from Chiang Mai in two olive oil bottles wrapped in cloths and put in a saddlebag along with Cort's lunch. It was "well packed because sometimes the ponies run." Once proper dosages were determined, injections became the responsibility of leprosy patients themselves.

Ebbe Kornerup observed the injections sometime between 1922 and 1924. He described the routine as follows: "In order not to make too much of the operation, this is performed publicly in an open arbour. The box containing the miraculous medicine is brought in; the patient bares his arm or leg, the president of the settlement washes it clean with spirits of wine, then paints it with iodine, and the doctor makes the injection . . . things are taken calmly in order to reassure the patient."

Five acres of *Hydnocarpus* trees were planted before 1923 with the hope that they would one day make the asylum self-sufficient in chaulmoogra oil.

In March 1927, the Hays Memorial Clinic/Infirmary was added to the complex. It had no more than a dozen beds, but allowed the residents to gather for treatment. It became the headquarters for the medical staff, pharmacy, and chaulmoogra injections. The missionary doctors (Cort and McKean) began to hold regular clinics three times a week. Improved medical care and better housing probably combined to bring the death rate down. In 1927 it was reported to be 6 percent, but in 1930 dropped to 4 to 5 percent, a significant improvement over the first year when the death rate was 14 percent.

A temporary school was built near the athletic field for children with leprosy. Three Thai teachers had an enrollment of thirty-two pupils in 1922. A second school was opened for the healthy offspring of leprosy patients (called untainted children by McKean), neighborhood children, and the offspring of non-leprosy workmen of the asylum.

Utilizing his expert horsemanship, McKean journeyed to other provinces to find leprosy victims and spread the news of the asylum. In Lampang and Wiang Pa Pao, McKean paid bearers to carry crippled leprosy beggars to Koh Klang. The price for leading a leprosy patient on the fifteen-day horseback journey was six baht (three dollars, U.S.).

Financial Burdens Increase

McKean felt the financial burden created by the steady growth in numbers but added, "It is hard to say nay to those that come in their dire need." He cited current expenses of $300 U.S. per month in 1915 and appealed for more donations. As the census grew, the directors added a third sub-village on the south end of the island. A large dormitory was built, originally called Bethesda Cottage, housing thirty women. This building survives today as the office for the social welfare department.

During the first seven years, the asylum population doubled every two years, peaking in 1914 and 1915 when an average of thirty residents were added annually. This was followed by a six-year deceleration attributed to high attrition rates and restored health due to chaulmoogra treatment. "Their improved physical condition begets the desire to get out and begin life again," states a report.

In fact, cures were rare. Only a small fraction (two of thirty in 1917) was cured when they left the asylum. Some left from discontent. The painful chaulmoogra injections were probably not a factor, since the treatment was voluntary. McKean attributed the monotonous life of the asylum as a reason, but the serious problem of overcrowding that arose in years of rapid growth seems to have been the most plausible explanation. In 1916, for example, there were accommodations for 130 patients, but the number of residents increased to 178. Two years later, many were housed in bamboo huts, since the permanent structures were full. The asylum simply could not raise funds and build

housing fast enough. The situation improved in the early 1920s when the Mary L. Stoner Village, consisting of forty-eight new wooden, double-occupancy cottages, was dedicated.

At the dedication of cottages, Mabel Cort stated, "They are very simple but complete. They are of wood with tiled roof. They are painted gray and are cemented underneath so that the drainage is good and easy to clean." The front room served as a bedroom while the back room served as a kitchen.

A fence separated women and men's sections. With men outnumbering women by three to one, the women attracted more attention than the conservative missionaries liked, resulting in a decision to move them.

Chaa Sua Hong was a wealthy Chinese merchant who had made a fortune through gambling in Bangkok. Cort's biographer, S. A. Schreiner, wrote how Dr. Cort "persuaded the Chinese gentleman that he would acquire more of the additional merit a man in his position

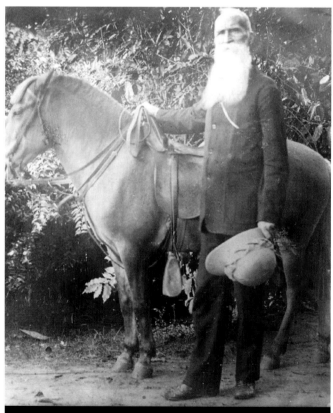

McKean often traveled by horse to find leprosy victims.

Chaulmoogra Oil

Imbedded in Indian folklore is a story of Rama, king of Benares, who cured himself and his bride, Piya, deep in a forest by eating the fruit and leaves of the kalaw tree. The belief in this miraculous cure was passed down for more than two thousand years. The kalaw tree was identified with "chaulmoogra," the Indian vernacular for the trees of genus *Hydnocarpus*. The name "chaulmoogra" gained acceptance for the drug produced from *Hydnocarpus* trees. Chaulmoogra was brought back to China after an ambassador's trip to Cambodia in 1295–1297 and was indicated as a possible cure for leprosy by Chu Chen-heng (1281–1358) although he disapproved of its use because of the irritating effect on the stomach.

In 1853, Professor F. J. Mouart at the Bengal Medical College Hospital in West India experimented on a leprosy patient with the god-king Rama's miraculous cure. He subsequently reported his patient's rapid response to the chaulmoogra seeds. This paved the way for disciplined testing of various preparations and administration methods. The drug gained attention in the U.S. in 1907, when Dr. Isadore Dyer of Tulane University reported successful use at the Indian Camp Plantation near Carville, Louisiana. An oral dose at that time might have been a capsule containing eight to ten drops, or up to thirty drops, if tolerated.

Chaulmoogra is fairly toxic. Put into water, it kills fish. Mixed with mouse chow and given to mice, it causes them to lose weight and die within a few weeks. Human doses were seldom high enough to kill people, but from the beginning, chaulmoogra use was limited by the adverse taste and the nausea and giddiness that followed consumption.

In the Philippines, it was found that only one out of three hundred leprosy cases could tolerate oral chaulmoogra. The drug had already been given experimentally by hypodermic needle when Dr. Victor Heiser and his Filipino worker, Mercado, introduced an improved solution of chaulmoogra oil for injection in 1910 and modified the preparation over the next ten years.

Initial reports from Thailand were also favorable. In 1916, E. C. Cort reported, "The aches and pains which had been constantly present heretofore, began to disappear, their appetites improved, and they gained in strength." Within three months the results looked good enough to send out a call for patients to come for treatment. By nine months, about two-thirds of the men, women, and children in the asylum were taking the weekly injections and Cort was sending news of his promising results to doctors overseas. At one year, he was starting to send some of the patients home, believing that the chaulmoogra had cured them.

Early enthusiasm gave way to sober reservations. By 1919, Chiang Mai doctors were no longer speaking of chaulmoogra as a cure, but merely a treatment that diminished some symptoms. Four years later, only 25 percent of the patients were willing to take the injections. Chaulmoogra oil treatment went out of fashion when the sulphonamides came into vogue in the late 1940s and early 1950s. Since the drug had no other medicinal use, it became obsolete. Yet, for at least thirty-five years, it was the mainstay of leprosy therapy. There is no clinical use of chaulmoogra oil in medicine today. Stately chaulmoogra trees (H. *anthelmintica* spec.) that were planted in the days of McKean still dot the landscape of the McKean Rehabilitation Center today.

needed by helping the mission curtail the birth of leprous babies. Chaa Sua Hong supplied enough money to move the women's quarters to the north end of the island, a good mile away from their amorous gentleman friends."

Administering the Growing Village

With the men and women separated, the directors decided the time had come to enforce a code of discipline. Nai Dobphromin Chaiworasin had been treated at Koh Klang and had become a Christian. He was asked to serve as a housefather. This decision was a stroke of great fortune, for by all accounts, Nai Dobphromin was a natural leader, wise and honest—just the sort of man for the job. He became superintendent for the men's village while an older couple, Ui Kham and Ui Moi were responsible for the women's village.

When Nai Dobphromin arrived, they had a community meeting and announced all of the rules by which the inhabitants would be expected to abide. He was entrusted with the arbitration of all disputes and arranging all community business decisions. At about the same time, new wooden cottages were opened and allocated to those who had shown good conduct.

Each village chose a headman by election. A secretary and an assistant secretary were also designated. Approximately thirty to forty guards, known as "policemen" (*damruij*) were

Nai Dobphromin Chaiworasin

added with five different rankings. Their duty was to keep the peace at Koh Klang.

The staff, almost entirely composed of leprosy patients, was divided into seven departments:

1. Religious
2. Personnel
3. Medical
4. School for children
5. Purchasing
6. Animal husbandry: pigs, ducks, and chickens
7. Maintenance/Forestry

The foundation for a meritocracy was laid and this system of self-government continues in large part to the present day.

Raising Funds for a Growing Program

As the population at the asylum boomed, McKean meticulously went about raising money. Equipped with a movie camera, he filmed the plight of leprosy victims and the new life they experienced at the asylum. These were silent movies, shown to church groups while a speaker read an accompanying text.

To illustrate the growth of the Koh Klang program, in 1908 there were three cottages and six adults. Twenty-two years later, at the McKeans's retirement, there were more than five hundred inhabitants (350 leprosy patients, the rest presumably non-leprosy relatives and employees); 143 buildings including 116 cottages, 9 dormitories, a church, an impressive administration building, a recreation center, a school, a sewing factory, and a tool and furniture factory. There was also a road for most of the island and a form of self-government based on the familiar village headman system. Film footage from H. M. King Rama VII's visit in 1927 shows the asylum looking the picture of neatness and space with all buildings decorated with European-looking white trim and the lanes cordoned by white picket fences.

From Institution to the Countryside

Chiang Mai Leper Asylum alumni gathered others around themselves for treatment. Some former patients built houses near each other. The only aid given to these people was rudimentary medicines. The presence of uninhabited forests made possible the spontaneous evolution of leprosy villages without conflicting with their neighbors. Leprosy homesteaders were permitted to stake their claim after three years of occupancy.

The people grew their own crops and lived like other villagers, except they were generally exempt from paying taxes or performing corvée labor. They did not visit outside villages except for trading purposes. Those who were crippled often went out begging, sometimes organizing themselves into groups to arrange transportation and begging venues. They begged for rice at residences and for money at marketplaces.

In the late 1920s and 1930s, there was an emphasis on nurturing villages and providing shelter rather than medical treatment. Forty-seven leprosy villages were started or supported in the following provinces: Nan, Chiang Rai, Phrae, Lampang, Mae Hong Son, Lamphun, Tak, Sukhothai, Pitsanulok, and Chiang Mai (which had eighteen villages, the most of any province involved). More than half of these leprosy villages no longer exist or have been taken over by the Thai government.

The McKean Era Reaches Its Twilight

By 1927, the McKeans were approaching the end of their missionary career. McKean had given up clinical medicine entirely, focusing all of his efforts on the leprosy asylum. In 1930, he attended the Far Eastern Society for Tropical Medicine Meeting in Bangkok. After the meeting, he invited all sixty of the attendees to visit the Chiang Mai Leper Asylum. They were impressed and declared it a model institution. That was his swan song.

The 1948 annual meeting overwhelmingly approved renaming the Chiang Mai Leper Asylum as the McKean Leper Home to honor the McKeans and their son, J. Hugh McKean. Today, it is known as the McKean Rehabilitation Center and Hospital, a service branch of the Church of Christ in Thailand. This institution has pioneered the integration of leprosy and non-leprosy disabled people into hospital-based and community-based rehabilitation programs. Visitors are welcome.

Behind the Legend: The McKeans as People

James McKean was remembered by colleagues as "likeable, quiet, and unassuming." The years no doubt mellowed him, but there is an appealing sense of humility in his writings, which make sparing reference to his own formidable accomplishments in combating infectious diseases while heaping generous praise on his Thai colleagues. This humility of spirit undoubtedly helped him succeed in organizing the efforts of several hundred workers in his leprosy and smallpox programs.

McKean, Chantah, and other Thai Christians who helped found the Koh Klang Hospital were motivated by a desire to spread the Gospel. He translated First and Second Corinthians into the northern dialect and helped to foster no less than four churches: Suebnathitam Church,

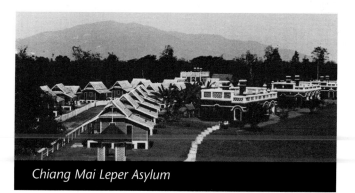

Chiang Mai Leper Asylum

Pete the Pig

Wilbur Chapman, the ten-year-old son of missionary parents who chaired the White Cloud (Kansas) Auxiliary, became a friend of "Uncle Will" Danner, then executive director of the American Leprosy Missions. In 1913, Wilbur saw Danner off at the railway station at 3:00 A.M. As they parted, Danner gave young Wilbur three silver dollars to use as he wished.

Wilbur knew how keenly disappointed his mother was that her campaign to raise $250 to support leprosy work in Siam, as portrayed in a public program by Dr. J. W. McKean, had fallen short by twenty-five dollars. With these three dollars, Wilbur purchased a piglet and raised it to maturity, hoping to fulfill his mother's goal. His friends joined in the excitement. They named the pig "Pete."

When the day came for "this little piggy to go to market" the selling price was twenty-five dollars! Excited, Wilbur sent the money to Uncle Will.

Danner shared the story with staff of the widely read *Sunday School Times*. The editor promptly installed a piggy bank in his office and published the story in his paper. What at first seemed to be an inspirational story became a new method of fundraising. Pete the Pig has taken on epic proportions. Like the lad in the biblical story of the feeding of the five thousand, this simple selfless deed has raised literally millions of dollars and helped to educate many about leprosy. A monument with a plaque showing Wilbur with his Pete the Pig stands in White Cloud, Kansas, today.

—Edgar Stoesz

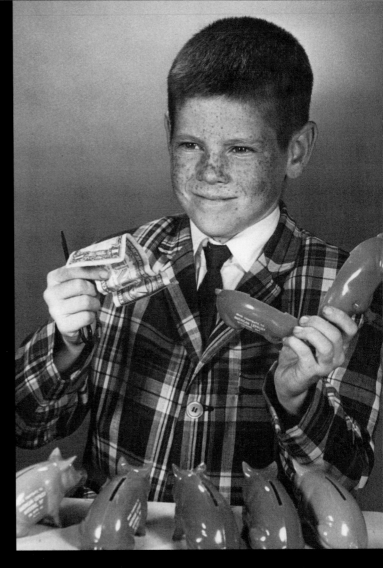

Above: A Sunday school child happily displays the contents of his "Pete" bank. Below: Pete the Pig bank

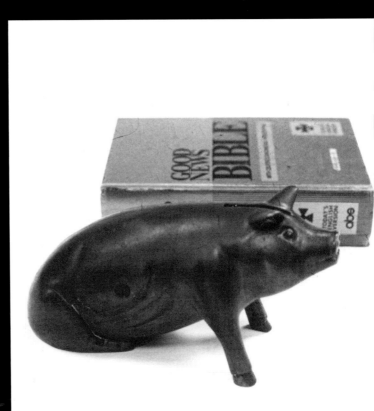

Ban Den Church, Mae Phu Kha parish, and, of course, the Koh Klang Church (now known as Santhitham Church).

McKean viewed leprosy as infectious and incurable, and believed that quarantine was an effective control measure, divinely justified in the laws of Moses. He testified before the U.S. Senate Committee on Public Health and Quarantine in 1916, and urged the quarantine of American leprosy victims. This hearing resulted in the first federal leprosy hospital in the United States, which opened in February 1921 at the Indian Camp Plantation, near Carville, Louisiana. The non-quarantined leprosy patients of Chiang Mai once collected an offering for leprosy sufferers in Carville. McKean's hope that the king of Siam would segregate the care of all leprosy sufferers did not come to pass.

Botany appears to have been one of McKean's hobbies. He promoted the idea of communal gardens in asylums. At least one field trip was made with noted botanist Dr. Arthur Kerr. The two wrote a paper on chaulmoogra oil–producing trees. The flower *Garcinia mckeaniana Craib* was named in McKean's honor.

Incongruous with his generally meek persona was McKean's penchant for speed; his galloping horseback escapades were legendary. When he upgraded to a Ford, his attraction to breakneck speed was unabated. Dr. E. M. Dodd recalled meeting him on a very rough road, steering the car with his left hand, while administering interval dabs of chloroform to a patient on the back seat with the other hand. McKean once fell asleep at the wheel on a return trip from Lamphun, and was only awakened by the jolt of stones at the side of the road. Dodd added, "He sang all the rest of the way home to keep awake."

Dr. Boonchom Ariwongse remembers calling on McKean at his Chiang Mai home. Boonchom had a boil in his groin and asked McKean to examine it. The venerable, gray-haired doctor, with one bad eye and his head cocked to one side, spoke in the old Northern Thai dialect, using the now archaic words *"gu"* and *"mung"* meaning "me" and "you." On the house porch and with no anesthesia handy, McKean lanced the abscess. Despite the pain, Boonchom thanked him, whereupon McKean replied: "You are the only one who has ever thanked me for doing something like that!"

A Fond Farewell

Having built up the American Hospital, vaccine laboratory, and leprosy asylum, the McKeans retired from more than forty-one years of service in Chiang Mai on March 10, 1931. McKean was honored by King Rama VII with the Order of the White Elephant (second class) and the Order of the Crown of Siam (third class), a double honor extended to only one other missionary, the Reverend William Harris, DD.

The McKeans took their final leave from Koh Klang after a church service. People lined up along the road for three quarters of a mile and threw flowers at the passing car. Dr. E. M. Dodd wrote, "It was hard for them to leave—he finally broke down at the gate when a group of lepers began to sing 'God Be with You.'"

While it took forty-two days to reach Chiang Mai by boat when they arrived in 1890, they departed in 1931 aboard the Royal Siamese Railway's *Bangkok-Chiang Mai Express* train, making the trip from Chiang Mai to Bangkok in twenty-six hours.

They resettled in California, first in Berkeley and then in Claremont, the home of their daughter, Kate. World War II denied the McKeans a final return visit. McKean was in waning health during his last dozen years in Thailand. Despite being laid low by bouts of overwork and dengue fever, troubled by tuberculosis and a bad heart, and blind in one eye since 1925, he enjoyed a long retirement in America. He continued to speak and raise funds on behalf of the work to which they had given their lives. James McKean died peacefully on February 9, 1949, at the age of eighty-eight, and was buried at Oak Park Cemetery in Claremont.

Laura McKean had many accomplishments of her own. As an entomologist, she found one new species of bees and three or four new moths and butterflies, all of which were given her name. She also made numerous Bible translations into the northern Thai script and English translations of Northern Thai folklore. Around 1915, however, she began to suffer poor health. In 1921, she went to the U.S. for treatment of what was thought to be a life-threatening case of oral cancer. She, nonetheless, outlived her husband by six weeks.

James McKean's contributions in building up the American Hospital have been over-shadowed by the achievements of his successor, Dr. E. C. Cort, who transformed it into McCormick Hospital, as it is known today. Likewise, McKean's diligence in spreading smallpox vaccination throughout Northern Thailand is nearly forgotten. It was McGilvary, founder of the American Presbyterian Mission in 1867, who foresaw what would be McKean's legacy. Shortly after the birth of the asylum, and shortly before his own death, McGilvary wrote: "It may be that the great work now enlisting Dr. McKean's sympathy and his strenuous efforts—the establishment of a leper colony and hospital, and the amelioration of the condition of that unfortunate class—may be the one with which his name will be most intimately associated." And so it is.

ABOUT THE AUTHOR

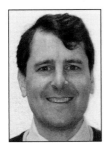

*D*r. Ted R. Brown grew up in Sacramento, California. He attended the University of California and graduated from Harvard Medical School in 1989. While in medical school, he studied care for the elderly in Japan with a Paul Dudley White Fellowship. That kindled his interest in Asia.

Brown completed a residency in physical medicine and rehabilitation at the University of Washington. During his residency and for one year following, he studied nerve damage and Hansen's disease at the McKean Rehabilitation Center in Chiang Mai, Thailand. In 1994, Brown became a full-time medical officer at McKean with a medical license provided by the Thai Ministry of Health. He stayed at McKean until 2002, working and living at the site of Dr. James McKean's legendary achievements.

After his 2002 return to the United States, Brown obtained a masters in public health at U.C. Berkeley. He is currently the multiple sclerosis clinical fellow at the University of Washington; and along with wife, Joy, he enjoys getting reacquainted with the Northwest.

Chapter 3

Congo: Featuring Eugene and Julia Kellersberger (1926–1945)

by Winifred Kellersberger Vass

Eugene Roland Kellersberger was almost not born. His mother, Helen Matern Kellersberger, wrote of his birth: "I was in labor forty-eight hours and feared toward the end that the baby was dead. Every time the labor pains came, he crawled back under my heart and I prayed, 'If this child is ever born, he must be used of God for a special purpose.'"

When Mrs. Holman, the midwife, saw that Mrs. Kellersberger was unable to deliver, she sent someone on horseback to call Dr. Christian. Upon his arrival the doctor bound towels about the mother's body to push the baby into position and forced the labor. It was none too soon. Mrs. Kellersberger's strength was completely spent. Both mother and baby came perilously close to dying.

The chosen name was that of the greatest of German heroes, Prince Eugene of Savoy. Even as an adult, Dr. Kellersberger remembered the gentle touch of his mother's hand on his cheek, as she said in a soft voice, "Prince Eugene, my noble knight!" She had the strong, intuitive conviction that this child was destined to be a knight of a different sort, who would do battle in another kind of war, against an enemy more than human.

As a child, Kellersberger idolized Getulius Kellersberger, his Swiss engineer grandfather. He listened raptly to the accounts of his nine-month voyage in 1849 and 1850 from New York City around Cape Horn to San Francisco, California, to join his brother Rudolf, the Swiss

consul. Getulius Kellersberger's first major employment in the United States was that of engineer for the City of Oakland.

While Eugene Kellersberger was general secretary of the American Leprosy Missions (1941–1953), he was a featured speaker in Oakland. He was taken to the city hall where he signed the guest register. Upon seeing the signature, the guard exclaimed, "Why, that's the same name as is on the city map of Oakland under glass in the mayor's office upstairs!" Kellersberger was taken immediately to meet the mayor and to see with his own eyes his grandfather's original map/plan of the city!

In 1924, Eugene Kellersberger penned an interesting summary of his own boyhood:

> During all the days of my boyhood till I was eighteen years old, my father had a general store, post office, gristmill and cotton gin, as well as a farm—in fact, all of this *was* Cypress Mill, Texas.

> As a whole, my boyhood was happy and never full of hard labor as I saw many other boys have to do. My life was more varied, the store and the post office being the center of a large community. It was a German-American community, mixed with Americans. There were no churches within ten to fifteen miles and there was no active religious life there, although

my father, raised a Catholic, and my sweet mother, granddaughter of a German Lutheran minister, were honest, truth loving, wonderful people.

As a boy, I had a horse, a gun and enjoyed swimming and fishing, especially on Sundays. I loved to read both German and English literature, George Eliot being my favorite author. I learned to speak both languages equally well. I always had a hunger for education and often begged my father to send me away to Austin. I was always ahead in the little country school and never quite fitted in.

At fifteen years I finally succeeded in persuading my father to let me go away to school in Austin. There I went—a green country boy who had never before ridden on a train, who put on long pants and shoes for the first time the day I left. I was traveling alone and dropped my baggage check behind the radiator in all the excitement of the seventy-five mile trip. I arrived in the city of Austin, awed and timid. There at the Whitis Academy I had three very important years of my life. It took that time to change me from an awkward country boy into something else. It took me that long to get away from some of the influences of the area where I had grown up and to gain for the first time a religious consciousness.

Kellersberger's third year at the Whitis Academy was without doubt his most interesting. Not only did he find his school subjects more absorbing, but there was also a new girl in his class! The name of Edna Helena Bosché was a welcome addition to the roster of the senior class of 1906. She had been a Whitis student from 1901 to 1903 and so was no stranger to the student body (even if she was to Kellersberger). The fact that this merry, outgoing lass, so pretty with the big pink bow in her dark hair, shared his

birth date, August 6, 1888, gave him a warm, personal pride and joy in her presence.

Shortly after classes began in the fall of 1905, Kellersberger's friend, Seth Hastings, persuaded him to attend Dr. Penick's Sunday school class for young men at the Highland Presbyterian Church. This was a critical turning point in Kellersberger's life. He was so impressed that he joined the class on the spot, rarely missing a Sunday after that. This was also the church of which Edna Bosché and her family were members, her father having given the original lots on which the sanctuary was built.

On June 6, 1906, Kellersberger was baptized in the Highland Presbyterian Church by Dr. Robert F. Kirkpatrick. He joined the church against his parents' wishes, for they were disturbed about his decision, being uncertain what "being a Presbyterian" meant. But Kellersberger was filled with a glad assurance that what he was doing was absolutely right for him. He wrote on that date: "Now I belong to *God!*"

Making a Medical Missionary

In the fall of 1907, the Phil Bosché family invited Kellersberger to share their home for as long as he was a student at the University of Texas at Austin. As Edna's Whitis classmate and sweetheart, and a member of their church, they knew him well. He was only too glad to accept!

Kellersberger enrolled for his freshman year at the University of Texas. Very early one morning, Edna Bosché came upon him reading her father's Bible in the most secluded corner of the Bosché family library. So engrossed was he that he did not hear her enter the room. Startled, he looked up from the depths of the big leather armchair, a guilty expression on his earnest, open face. He had never had a chance to read the Bible before. He was wondering if he could borrow this one for a little while each morning; he was curious to know what it said.

Being caught red-handed with a Bible was the beginning of a lifetime habit. He was given his own Bible and, from then on, every day for an hour before breakfast, he and his sweetheart read and studied it together. If they were apart, they read the same agreed upon passages, at the same hour of each day. It was in this atmosphere of warm acceptance, undergirded by intercessory prayer and deep spiritual concern, that Kellersberger's faith matured and became strong and vital. It is little wonder that, in the years that followed, he was fond of saying, "I found Jesus Christ in the Bosché home."

Edna Bosché and Kellersberger saw little of each other during the academic sessions of 1908 to 1910, for she was in Chicago, a student at the Moody Bible Institute. Kellersberger continued to live with the Boschés where he was a totally accepted member of the family circle. The engaged couple kept in touch through weekly letters and in their common daily Bible study hour.

During the summer of 1909, Kellersberger accompanied the Bosché family to the World Missions Conference, sponsored by the Executive Committee of Foreign Missions of the Presbyterian Church, in Montreat, North Carolina. Edna Bosché was not with them, for her study program at Moody continued through the summer months.

Montreat is located in a quiet, wooded cove of the Smoky Mountains, near Asheville. It was there that Kellersberger had long talks with the famous medical missionary to Korea, Dr. Wylie Hamilton Forsythe, who had been brutally beaten and left for dead by a band of vicious Korean outlaws.

Amid the sun-dappled rhododendron thickets, with the music of the nearby rushing mountain stream flowing over the rocks, Forsythe put his arm around the shoulders of the young pre-med student from Texas and prayed aloud for him from an overflowing heart. It was then that Kellersberger made the personal decision to give his life in medical missionary service in Africa.

By the end of his junior year in 1910, Kellersberger's natural gifts in anatomy, biology,

and chemistry were apparent. He was named student assistant in the University of Texas Biology Department for his senior year.

Kellersberger began his studies at the Washington University School of Medicine in St. Louis, Missouri in October, 1911. At the close of his first year, he ranked first in his class and was awarded the Gill Prize in Anatomy.

Edna and Eugene Kellersberger were married on June 18, 1912, in a quiet ceremony in the Bosché home. Mother Bosché was very frail and died soon after the wedding.

Dr. Kellersberger graduated with his degree in medicine in 1915. His gold Alpha Omega Alpha key hung proudly from his watch chain. He served his internship at Kansas City General Hospital. The physician who made the deepest impression on the young intern was Dr. Arthur Emmanuel Hertzler, a Mennonite of horse-and-buggy fame. Unlike present-day highly specialized residencies, there were rotating internships covering two intensive months each in internal medicine, surgery, pediatrics, and obstetrics. Ward study of patients was also in operation in Kansas City hospitals. Individual patients were assigned to interns for history, examination, diagnoses, and treatment.

Hertzler's professional contributions to Kellersberger were his surgical anesthesiological techniques. He was the first doctor to introduce into the

Eugene Kellersberger

Leonard Wood Memorial
(American Leprosy Foundation)

The Leonard Wood Memorial (LWM) grew out of the visionary humanitarian concern of Major General Leonard Wood. On becoming the United States governor-general of the Philippines in 1921, Wood visited the leprosarium on Culion Island, which had seven thousand segregated leprosy patients. Overwhelmed by their plight, he vowed to work for their improvement.

Wood, a physician, sought the counsel of H. W. Wade, professor of pathology at the University of the Philippines in Manila, because Wade was conducting research on leprosy. Persuaded that the path to a better understanding and treatment of leprosy was through scientific research, Wade made relevant proposals. Wood was sympathetic with Wade's convictions but unable to obtain government funds to support research.

While Wade and his wife were disappointed, they were not discouraged. In 1925, the indomitable Mrs. Wade went to the United States and "knocked the doors of many important people." Her persistence was eventually instrumental in forming the American Committee for the Eradication of Leprosy with the support of such prominent statesmen, financiers, and industrialists as Charles Evans Hughes, William Howard Taft, W. Cameron Forbes, and Eversley Childs. By 1928, endowment goals were achieved and The Leonard Wood Memorial for the Eradication of Leprosy was incorporated. A modern leprosy research laboratory was set up on Cebu Island and this became the focal point of LWM, while work continued at Culion.

The LWM has coordinated significant leprosy research and training on a worldwide basis. The International Leprosy Association (ILA) was established at an LWM-sponsored scientific meeting in 1931. LWM assumed responsibility for the ILA-sponsored International Journal of Leprosy until the 1970s, when it was replaced by ALM. In 1950 the LWM established the Leprosy Registry at the Armed Forces Institute of Pathology (Washington D.C.), which now contains the largest extant documented collection of clinical specimens on leprosy. LWM-supported activities in the broad field of leprosy research include epidemiology, chemotherapy, diagnosis, microbiology, and immunology.

Originally LWM established offices in New York and Washington, but now its headquarters are in Rockville, Maryland. For more than three-quarters of a century, LWM has been a valuable colleague with ALM in the campaign to conquer leprosy.

—**Dr. Wayne Meyers**

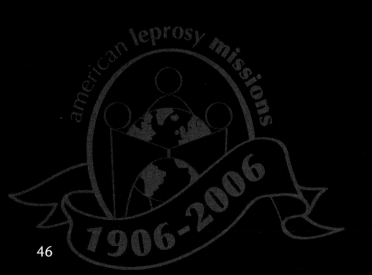

United States the use of cocaine in local anesthesia. Ether had been invented in 1846, followed by chloroform in 1872. Ether was considered safer and was given by the "drop method." After going to the mission field, Kellersberger trained his Congolese male nurses to do this extremely well.

The Crucible (1916–1923)

The Kellersbergers sailed for their first Belgian Congo mission assignment in October 1916. It was in the depth of World War I, before the United States had joined in the battle. All portholes and entryways of the sixteen-thousand-ton French liner *Lafayette* were carefully draped with heavy black cloth to prevent any chink of light from betraying the presence of a vessel to a lurking German raider.

Landing safely at Bordeaux, France, on November 13, the Congo-bound missionaries eagerly awaited the arrival of the *Afrique*, the oldest vessel of the line, which had long since been declared unseaworthy, and which would take them to Africa. So many ships had been sunk by the Germans that even the oldest had once again been pressed into service. God's protective hand was on the old vessel during the rough, month-long voyage to Matadi at the mouth of the Congo River. It arrived safely, but on the return voyage to Europe, it split in two and went to the bottom of the sea with no survivors.

Arriving at his first assigned post of Lusambo mission station, Kellersberger discovered that his daily clinic was housed in a twelve-by-twelve foot open shed with a grass roof. There was a three-by-five foot mud-walled enclosure at one end, where he stored his drugs and medical instruments. The carpenter's bench was his examination and operation table and a five-gallon kerosene drum was his sterilizer. Patients began to pour in from as far as two hundred miles away.

The diseases that Kellersberger encountered at Lusambo were legion. Among those listed is the first mention of leprosy and sleeping sickness, the two diseases that he eventually treated by the thousands.

One morning soon after his arrival, a sixty-foot, nearly three-foot-wide, dugout canoe landed at the Mission's Sankuru River beach, manned by sixteen muscular boatmen with hand-carved wooden paddles. Rev. Wilson of the English Brethren Mission thirty miles downriver had been attacked by a hooded buffalo; a surgeon was needed immediately. The marvelous rhythm and perfectly synchronized movement of those powerful oarsmen, together with the staccato voice and persistent tapping of the leader's stick on the side of the boat, brought Dr. Kellersberger's surgical aid to Wilson in record time.

During the Kellersbergers's first furlough in the United States (1921–1922), the doctor received permission from the Mission Board to go to England and take the three-month certificate course in tropical medicine at the London School of Tropical Medicine. God's amazing providence in this became evident a few months later when Edna was bitten by an infected tsetse fly during a nine-hundred-mile Congo and Kasai riverboat journey. Shortly after returning to Bibanga Station, she began running a low-grade fever and having headaches.

On August 26, 1921, Kellersberger, using his microscope, found trypanosomes in a thick drop of her blood. They had no choice but to return as soon as possible to London, England, the only place where treatment was available.

Kellersberger took their two daughters to stay with family in the U.S. while his wife was in the London Hospital for Tropical Diseases for eight months. She was one of the first patients to be successfully treated by Sir Patrick Manson and Dr. Carmichael Low, who cured her of sleeping sickness with Bayer 205. After a brief visit with his kin in Switzerland, the couple returned to the United States. For four precious months the family was together. How the Kellersbergers reveled in their joyous reunion with their two daughters!

On January 28, 1923, Dr. Egbert Smith, executive secretary of the Foreign Missions Committee of the Presbyterian Church, made a special trip to talk to the Kellersbergers. News had come that Dr. Stixrud, the only doctor on the Belgian Congo mission field, had sleeping sickness.

"Eugene, if you feel Edna is now well enough for you to leave, would you be willing to return alone to the Congo immediately?" Dr. Smith asked. Together on their knees, the Kellersbergers made the painful decision that he would return for a two-year term, the length of time that his wife's London doctors felt that she should remain in a temperate climate before attempting to return to tropical Africa.

For the eighth time in a little over two years, Kellersberger made a transatlantic crossing. The few days that he spent in London were medically exciting. He had lunch with Dr. Manson-Bahr and visited Dr. Carmichael Low, learning there were now six cured cases of sleeping sickness, all treated with Bayer 205. From London, Kellersberger went to Germany where he spent a week in the laboratories of Farben Fabriken in Leverkusen, a suburb of Cologne. Speaking his native German, Kellersberger carefully studied the manufacturing process of Bayer 205.

In Brussels, he had an important conference with Dr. A. Broden, the Belgian *Medecin en Chef,* obtaining letters of introduction to the Belgian Medical Service in Elisabethville. He was also given a letter from the colonial minister to the governor of Katanga Province, granting him permission to spend a month in Elisabethville, doing research on African sleeping sickness.

These crucial weeks that Kellersberger spent in Elisabethville in 1923 turned his medical service sharply in the direction of public health. He was given the full status of a *Medecin Agree,* an officially recognized Belgian Colonial Service Doctor. Kellersberger's experience in sleeping sickness control was excellent preparation for the work he would soon be doing in the field of leprosy.

At 10 A.M. on May 22, 1923, Kellersberger on his bicycle, followed by his trotting caravan of baggage-carriers, ascended the last long hill up to Bibanga Mission Station. The local population knew of his imminent arrival. The communication drums and signal whistles had been sending the message over the hills since early morning. All along the trail, during the last hour of travel, jubilant villagers rushed to join the caravan, racing alongside the chanting carriers, escorting their doctor triumphantly back onto the Bibanga compound.

The first unit of the hospital plant had been completed during his furlough absence. As one in a dream, Kellersberger walked over the clean, white cement floor of the five-room administrative unit. He indicated which room would house the clinic, which the dispensary and the laboratory, and which was to be his private office. In a daze, he showed where he wanted the shelves and tables to be placed. On May 25, a dedication service was held with a large crowd present. The first clinic opened as soon as the service was over.

Then on November 5, 1923, Kellersberger received the shock of his life. In the middle of a hotly contested tennis match with missionary colleagues, a messenger handed him a telegram that read as follows:

REGRET TO REPORT THE SUDDEN DEATH OF MRS KELLERSBERGER OCTOBER 23. ADVISE KELLERSBERGER REMAIN ON THE FIELD. CHILDREN WITH MRS BROWN.
—Executive Committee of Foreign Missions

An African colleague insisted on spending the night with him. Kellersberger could not reconcile himself to stay on the field as instructed and proceeded to hurriedly make arrangements for the two-month return journey via Antwerp and New York. He knew the funeral had already taken place, but he was also concerned about the care of his two young daughters.

It was understandably a difficult time, but Kellersberger's return to continue his African medical mission calling was never in doubt. A measure of comfort came to him when, at the suggestion of Charles Lukens Huston, the lead donor of the Bibanga hospital asked that it be named in Edna's memory. A plaque on the hospital reads:

The Edna Kellersberger Memorial Hospital
Mamu Munanga

"Greater love has no man than this, to lay down his life for his friends."—John 15:13

Construit en 1923–1924

Edna Kellersberger's Bantu-language name, *Mamu Munanga*, means Beloved Mother.

During the first complete year of work at the Edna Kellersberger Memorial Hospital, Kellersberger held 17,599 consultations. One American doctor, assisted by one American nurse and fourteen Congolese nurses did ninety-three operations, all in a three-unit hospital with a thirty-bed capacity.

Diseases treated included 263 cases of subtertian malaria, hookworm (594), hernias (52), schitosomiasis (108), plus assorted cases of meningitis, leprosy, yaws, amoebic and bacillary dysentery, smallpox, goiters, and elephantiasis.

Operation for a Prince

On August 6, 1925, Kellersberger hosted Crown Prince Leopold of Belgium on an official visit. The day before the scheduled visit to observe Protestant medical work, a small woman, some thirty years of age, a mere skeleton, registered at the clinic. She could not speak, for out of her mouth protruded an epulis, a foul-smelling ulcerating tumor as big as an orange. It spread out against each cheek, down over her chin and pushed her nose up so that she could barely breathe. She could open her mouth just enough to push in a little food; she was starving to death.

Trust of the Unexplained

While grieving the tragic death of his wife, Kellersberger wrote the following in his prayer notebook:

Anew I dedicate my life, my all to Christ. The loveliest sweetest thing on earth He has taken away. She wanted me to be a *living sacrifice* for Christ in Africa. O Christ! I dedicate myself anew to Africa! The fellowship of His suffering is now so very real to me. I am being made conformable to His death for whom I have suffered the loss of all things. Oh God! Help me to bear the pain, the ache of her being gone! All life was so full of her—nothing I did without her! And now she is GONE! Such emptiness! Fill it with THYSELF! Replace what I have lost with THYSELF. Dear Lord! Though *He slay me, yet will I trust Him.* Let self be crucified and Christ enthroned in my life because of this experience.

—excerpt from *Doctor Not Afraid*

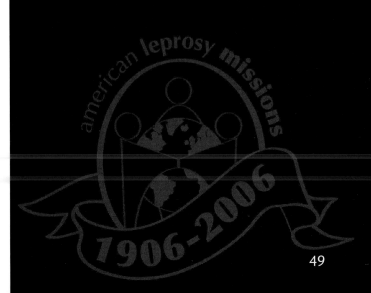

Watching the Prince's facial reaction to the sight and smell of this woman, Kellersberger thought, *God must have sent her to us precisely on this special day just to glorify His name.*

Crown Prince Leopold stared at her, then turned to Kellersberger and questioned, "Do you intend to operate on this woman?"

"Of course! That's why I'm here, to do this in Christ's name."

"I am on my way to Kabinda, but will come back through here day after tomorrow. When I return, I want to see this woman."

When the prince and his retinue returned to the hospital, she was waiting for him, holding in her hands the bottle that contained the tumor removed the day before. The bottle with its contents was presented to the prince, who took it back to Belgium, a unique souvenir of his visit to Bibanga. The Brussels daily newspaper, *Independence Belge,* published an account of the crown prince's experience.

The Scourge of Sleeping Sickness

From 1925 to 1928, Kellersberger was occupied with the control and eradication of African sleeping sickness (trypanosomiasis). He was superbly fitted for dealing with this disease by his wife's having had it. It became evident that only a small percentage of the population was coming voluntarily to be examined, with Kellersberger examining some seventeen thousand men, women, and children. Four hundred new cases were found in all stages of advancement.

Kellersberger was the only doctor on the American Presbyterian Congo Mission for long periods of time. Since he was responsible for caring for the personnel of five mission stations scattered over eighty-three thousand square miles of south-central Belgian Congo, there was always a long list of operative cases awaiting his attention!

But the doctor never forgot that he was an ordained minister as well as a physician. He regularly went without breakfast on Sunday mornings

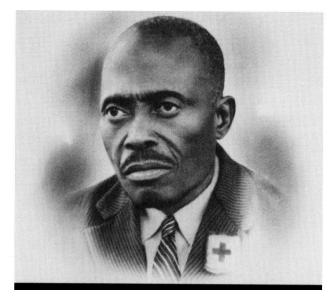

Samuel Lubilashi, head nurse of the Edna Kellersberger Memorial Hospital at Bibanga, 1920–1980. He was trained by Dr. Kellersberger to be his chief surgical assistant.

to have quiet time for sermon preparation. If he was not the designated preacher at the station church or hospital chapel, he was off on his bicycle to hold a service in some distant village. Every Sunday afternoon his cherished class of young men gathered on his front porch for a thoughtful, prayed-over Bible lesson, sometimes prepared at the cost of even more sleep.

A New Direction In Leprosy

Kellersberger married Miss Julia Lake Skinner in Mt. Berry, Georgia, on February 3, 1930. The busiest and most fulfilling years of his life were the last two terms, from 1930 through 1940. The cheerful, supportive presence of his outgoing, remarkably gifted new wife, Julia Lake, and his two beloved daughters, united again with him in a congenial family unit, provided a deeply satisfying base for a new, many-faceted ministry.

This decade of service, broken by one furlough in 1935–1936, was a crucial period of transition. During this time his interest and concerns shifted from general tropical medicine and surgery to specialization in Hansen's disease. These were also pivotal years of firsthand experience in organizational administration and fundraising, a direct result of the Great Depression and its effects on the work of the American Presbyterian Congo Mission.

In the very beginning of the medical work at Bibanga, Kellersberger often referred in his diaries to the ever-present group of leprosy sufferers, sadly eyeing him from under what came to be called "The Leper Tree." Over the years they came and went, camping for weeks, hopeful of some attention. A few left, returning to God-knew-where; others came, also hoping. Always some were there, stolidly waiting, day and night.

Finally, in 1929 the American Presbyterian Congo Mission was permitted "to explore the possibility of a pilot leprosarium to be operated without cost to the Mission." The 1930 mission meeting approved leprosy work on the condition "that it be self-supporting as to feeding, housing and 50 percent of the drugs." The real break-through came in 1931, when the following actions were taken and a large red "A" for "Answered" was written across the pages of Kellersberger's prayer notebook.

Minute 31-500—Bibanga Camp approved, with Dispensary, Dormitory Unit, Church, School and Workshop.

Minute 31-700—The Executive Committee of Foreign Missions approves the application to the American Mission to Lepers, for support of leprosy work, Bibanga to be the pilot station for this work, $10,000 to be requested from the American Mission to Lepers.

By 1937 there were leprosaria on each of the five major stations of the American Presbyterian Congo Mission.

Choosing the Site for the Bibanga Leprosarium

An ideal location for the Bibanga Leprosarium was found three miles from Bibanga Mission Station. It was a wide, level semi-circular plateau overlooking a fertile valley full of springs, lakes, and patches of forest. There was ample room for many small gardens and fields.

When Kellersberger and the local Belgian administrator met with the area tribal chief to discuss the mission's request for a location of the new leprosarium, it became apparent that there was a problem. Part of the land being requested had been an ancient tribal burial ground. A white-barked "spirit tree" had grown to huge proportions, a landmark indicating the presence of ancient ancestral spirits.

The chief and his elders refused to grant this hallowed area, but they did offer in its place a better plot of agricultural ground adjoining the ancestral land. The chief willingly granted the American Presbyterian Congo Mission a concession of fifty-four hectares of his tribal land on the plateau for the leprosy village itself. The exact location of the dispensary, the head nurse's residence, the church, the school, and the carpenter's workshop were decided upon and carefully surveyed. By October, the first streets had been measured and laid out, as well as the exact location for the native houses for the eagerly waiting residents.

Kellersberger kept daily diaries for fifty years. His brief diary entries record the progress of the construction work that was so joyously and vigorously launched at this time:

1930
October 5—Work at Leper Camp started. Building the first 40 Leper Houses, the Nurse's Residence, Pharmacy and the Lazaret (a quarantine station to house contagious cases).
December 26—Sixty Lepers already here!
December 28—Held our first Sunday service. I preached to the Lepers.

1931
January 1—Gave gift of meat to all residents.
January 6—122 now in the camp.
January 9—Happy Day! Leper Camp officially opened.

Never Afraid to Touch

Though busy with his role as head of the expanding American Leprosy Missions, Dr. Kellersberger always had his antenna out for someone in need. So, while living in New York, he followed a lead to what he first thought was an abandoned saloon. There greeting him was what he knew instinctively was a victim of leprosy. She was a middle-aged woman of Mexican descent with a badly disfigured face and hands. In the cold, bare room he spoke to her. She answered in broken English. She knew she did not have long to live, but neither did she want to go to a government leprosarium.

"Has anyone prayed with you?" asked Dr. Kellersberger. She gave him a long, searching look. It did not matter that she was Catholic and he was Protestant. He told her that Christ died for her sins and that He, the great Physician, was the only one able to help her both physically and spiritually.

Then he laid hands on her, spoke a blessing, and prayed for her. As he did so, kneeling beside her on the bare, damp floor, he recalled the words from Psalm 142:4, "No man cared for my soul."

Suddenly she broke into a torrent of tears. After some time she gained her composure and said in broken English, "Doctor, no money on earth can ever pay you for what you have done for me today."

January 10—First stage of construction of Leper Camp has been finished! A joy to see these poor, finger-less and toe-less people go to their Camp homes!

January 11—Sunday—The first official worship service was held under the palm trees. Sixty lepers were seated on long fallen logs. I preached on "Touching Jesus!" A happy lot they are now! They have "Come from death to life!"

January 12—Still more Lepers coming in! The camp is growing! 27 houses are now occupied. Happy work!

January 14—New stick-and-grass church now going up. More Lepers pouring in. Having to fight them off to keep control. Poor fellows! It's hard for them to wait!

January 17—99 Lepers in our church service this morning. Thank God! Our camp is getting pretty, too!

January 20—Fifty more Lepers crying to get into our camp. Full for the present. Sad! But I must keep things under control!

January 24—Every house has been taken. We are completely filled up and many more are trying to get in.

February 2—Leper camp now in full swing! We are putting up other buildings to house them.

February 8—Dedicated our new church today at the Leper camp, 146 present. I preached on "Heart Spots." There was a regular revival of response to my message! Many confessions of sin!

February 12—Held clinic all morning at the Leper camp. Getting it all organized fine!

March 1—Visitors again coming to see our camp. Leprosy + tuberculosis = BAD!

March 20—Have started our school! Stayed all day at the camp. Examined each patient for "swellings." Planted mango and papaya trees.

April 12—Sunday Service at the Leper camp. 178 present. Showed intense interest and attention. I gave my "Idol Sermon."

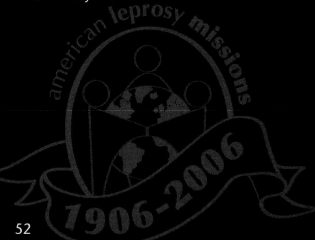

April 21—Our home board has given a 44 percent cut to us in our Mission funds! Depression years! God Help Us! He has! He is! He will!

April 23—Torrential rains caused land slide at the Leper camp spring in the valley. An 8-year-old boy was killed in the land slide. An avalanche of mud and dirt buried him.

April 24—Went to the camp tonight with our victrola. Played in the moonlight.

Principles for Maintaining a Successful Leprosarium

In 1939 Dr. Ernest Muir, secretary-treasurer of the International Leprosy Association (ILA) visited the leprosarium in Bibanga. Muir's common sense interpretation of each individual condition resulted in grouping leprosy into the following classes:

1. Neural [any leprosy affecting the nerves]
2. Mixed Cutaneous [a mixture of different skin lesions]
3. Tuberculoid [few skin lesions and very few bacilli in the tissues; the body's resistance is high]
4. Lepromatous [many skin lesions and many bacilli in the tissues; the body's resistance is low]
5. Borderline [in between, with some features of each type; immunologically unstable and can cause widespread nerve damage]

Segregation of all lepromatous cases with the leprosy village was deemed to be of extreme importance. Equally important was the separation of children from infected parents.

Muir believed that the rest of the leprosarium population should be categorized as follows:

1. Arrested [slowed]
2. Aborted [stopped in the early stages; remain rudimentary]
3. Inactive [quiescent; causing no trouble or symptoms]

4. Cured [the disease is absent; restored to health, soundness, or normality]

Using these classification techniques permitted the discharging of many patients, resulting in reducing the inpatient census from 500 to 325. "We were able to tell a large number that their disease was arrested, or quiescent, or inactive or cured. We also learned the great importance of segregating the lepromatous in their own part of the village. We learned the importance of separating children from their infected parents and the great importance of the improvement in their general health," Kellersberger wrote in 1939.

Muir observed that African leprosy was milder than in the Orient, with less open cases and fewer mutations. This was believed to be due to less crowding, less contact, and more balanced diet.

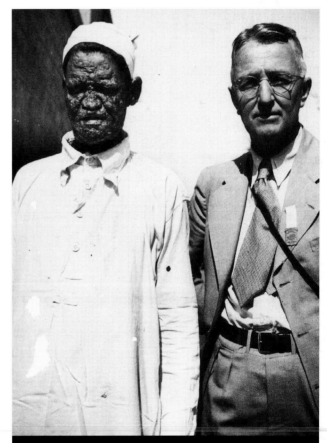

Leprosy patient with Dr. Eugene Kellersberger at the Cairo government leprosarium in 1938.

Pied Piper of the Leper Colony

He might not always be the first you saw when driving in the entrance to the Luebo Leprosarium, but he was certainly the first you heard.

His name was Kweta and for years he had been an inmate of the leprosy village administered a few miles from our station by the combined support of our mission and the Belgium colonial government and the American Leprosy Missions.

He was an ex-soldier, a crusty old veteran of the campaign of World War I—Belgian Congo troops were engaged against the Germans in East Africa. He had been a bugler and his most prized possession was an antiquated bugle, the kind that you see pictured in battle scenes of the 1800s, made of brass, all curled up like a ram's horn.

The sound of any approaching motor was the signal for him to snatch that worn, coppery instrument and start a lively march across the compound. He was the self-appointed welcoming committee, and visitors to the leprosarium were always greeted with a flourish of liquid bugle notes as they stepped down from the doctor's car. As they made their rounds of the colony, Kweta was always ahead, proudly blowing a musical "make-way," trailed Pied Piper-like by a happy crowd of the less crippled inmates, with visitors bringing up the rear.

Kweta's bugle was the symbol of hope restored when all hope was gone, a bugle blowing the sounds of the high triumph through village streets, walked only by the maimed.

Thank you, Lord, for Kweta's very special offering of a joyful noise. In heaven I'm sure He will have not only new feet but also a new horn.

—from *Thirty-One Banana Leaves*
by Winifred Kellersberger Vass

The International Leprosy Congress

In March 1938, Kellersberger received an invitation from Secretary of State Cordell Hull to represent the United States at the International Leprosy Congress in Cairo, Egypt. Mrs. Kellersberger convinced him that this was an honor worth cashing in his only life insurance policy, yielding eight hundred dollars, exactly enough to pay for a round-trip ticket.

Kellersberger drove to Kabalo, the nearest railroad point east of Bibanga. There, he boarded the wood-burning train for Albertville on Lake Tanganyika. Then came a cruise on a lake steamer from Albertville north to Kigoma in Tanganyika. From there, another train took him to Mwanza on Lake Victoria in Uganda.

On Friday, March 17, *Ceres*, the "flying boat," took the doctor from Kampala, Uganda, to Cairo, Egypt. Kellersberger described the dramatic landing on Lake Victoria as "an amazing sight. . . . like a great whale with wings, landing so gracefully on the water!"

After a 610-mile flight at an altitude of seven thousand feet over the papyrus swamps of the Upper Nile, the *Ceres* made a refueling stop at Malahal, Anglo-Egypt. It took off again in a cloud of spray, flying at an altitude of nine thousand feet at 150 mph! A landing was made in Khartoum, Sudan to spend the night.

The next day's flight included a breathtaking descent through a storm, circling to land on the Nile for refueling at Wadi Halfa. Motor boats handling the refueling had a terrible time! Finally, the *Ceres* was off again, flying over the tomb of Rameses and the three giant pharaohs hewn out of the cliff beside the Nile. The pilot flew very low to improve the view.

On March 20, Kellersberger met his friend, Dr. Ernest Muir, the Congress chairman, at Cairo University. He served as the chairman's German, French, and English interpreter throughout the conference. The opening session was in the Grand Opera House. Representatives of fifty-four nations sat on the stage, all robed in black academic gowns. "I sat very close to King Farouk," wrote Kellersberger, "he's a fine looking man!"

There were three-hour sessions morning and afternoon, with lectures given in one of six languages: Arabic, French, English, German, Spanish, and Italian. Subjects covered were "Classification of Leprosy Cases"; "Cultures of Leprosy"; "Treatment of Leprosy"; and "The Human Side of Leprosy." Kellersberger delivered his address on March 25.

A reception for one thousand people was given by King Farouk at Abadin Palace, with supper served at midnight. Of this occasion Kellersberger wrote: "Such display of wealth and pomp, such royal food and prodigal hospitality! It was an Arabian Night's scene in a fairy palace!"

The Chaulmoogra Oil Tree Plantation

Kellersberger became intrigued by experimenting with the effects of chaulmoogra oil on patients in his Bibanga leprosarium. In 1930 he ordered, by way of friends in Ceylon, "enough seed to start a large grove of the healing tree."

Kellersberger received a *pepiniere*, a whole portable nursery seedbed, of six hundred chaulmoogra oil trees, ready for planting. The first planting was done in January; the second, in April. By February of 1935, the flourishing trees were in flower. Hope was high—the long-awaited and prayed-for cure was in sight.

On July 24, 1936, Kellersberger recorded that the trees were bearing seed. A Belgian friend working at the nearby Katanda Cotonco post

donated a hand-operated press to extract oil from the chaulmoogra nuts. Kellersberger wrote:

> We get the best results with fresh, whole Chaulmoogra oil with 5 percent Creosote added. Two injections are given to one patient weekly, from 1 c.c. up to 10 c.c. per injection. A special feature of our colony is our thriving 1200-tree plantation of Chaulmoogra oil trees. The trees are now nine years old and have been bearing for four years. This is the only producing plantation in the Belgian Congo.

The Kellersbergers's last two years on the field were the most harried, uprooted, unpredictable years of their lives. The local population had come to rely on their services. At the same time, the approaching war left them with a deficit of qualified personnel. Drugs were no longer available from Europe, threatened by the German invasion. Currency problems abounded daily, making everyday commerce frustrating.

Returning late from a particularly difficult trip, Kellersberger found a letter awaiting him from Dr. Emory Ross, general secretary of the American Mission to Lepers. Ross had accepted another assignment and was now informing Kellersberger that the board had voted unanimously to invite him to be Ross's successor.

It was not a difficult decision. Noting that there were just eleven more operations in his operating record book, he said, "It's time for me to go home."

Emory Ross

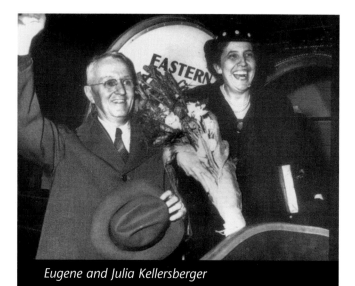
Eugene and Julia Kellersberger

As recorded in his diary:

The last Sunday at the camp was a happy and touching time, complete with flowers and songs. Church full to overflowing. Fine attention. No one wanted to leave after the service. Kept sitting. Opportunity to bring a real message: Christ is the same forever. (Heb 13:08) They must forget me, the transient human worker and depend on the never changing, eternal Head of all the work. Some of the women cried, "You are not afraid to touch us." So tired and happy.

Our final goodbye. As the car pulled out, great crowds came to see us off. Stopped at the leprosarium. What a send off. Very touching. Flowers and bouquets piled high all over the car. I did hate to leave them most of all.

Four months intervened between closing the Belgium Congo career and the beginning of a new career at the American Mission to Lepers headquarters in New York, soon to conclude its fourth decade. Fifty of these days were on the high seas early in World War II, as dangerous as the first crossing in 1916 on the unseaworthy *Afrique*.

Kellersberger, true to his nature, hit the ground running, with first a round of speaking engagements and then settling into his New York office. A modest apartment was found eight blocks from the office, decorated by Julia with a strong African motif. She served as the promotions secretary while Kellersberger served as general secretary. A constant theme in Kellersberger's diaries was "Sunshine in my coffee cup." Neighbors asked, "Are you the people who live in the apartment where so many people are coming and going?"

Kellersberger served as general secretary of the American Mission to Lepers from 1941 to 1953. In 1946, the Kellersbergers traveled to forty countries, visited sixty-five leprosy establishments (forty-two supported by AML), and saw more than thirty-five thousand people with Hansen's disease.

Seeing his approaching retirement, he asked a friend, Homer Rodeheaver (Billy Sunday's famous song leader), if he knew of any civilized place in the United Sates where he might make up for twenty-five years of lost fishing time. Rodeheaver replied, "Come be my neighbor on South Melbourne Beach in Florida."

And so it was that the Kellersbergers changed their residence and their vocation . . . a little. Both were still busy with speaking engagements and a heavy flow of visitors, though fishing was also on the weekly schedule. There were signs of diminished health; entries in the diaries were shorter and less frequent. One day, while fishing, with the beautiful sunset in sight, he breathed his last. Doctor Not Afraid had entered his eternal reward.

Since Eugene Kellersberger's death on July 28, 1966, much has happened in regard to the treatment of leprosy. He must be rejoicing in heaven over the breakthrough of multiple drug therapy (MDT). Both multiple-lesion (MB) and single-lesion (PB) patients are responding well to it! We pray God's blessings on every effort worldwide to minister to the victims of leprosy, the only disease that the Lord Jesus Christ specifically named during His life here on earth!

ABOUT THE AUTHOR

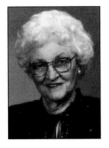

*W*inifred Kellersberger Vass was born in Lusambo, Belgium Congo, the daughter of Presbyterian missionary parents. Educated by her stepmother through high school years, Vass was often with her doctor father, either at the hospital or the leprosarium. She graduated in 1938 from Agnes Scott College with a degree in French and a teaching certificate. In June 1940 she married Rev. Lachlan C. Vass, son of another long term Congo missionary family.

Vass and her husband served with the American Presbyterian Congo Mission from 1940 to 1970, working primarily in literature development, publication, and editing journals in the Tshiluba language. She received a master's degree in journalism and communications from the University of Florida in 1971 where she also had conferred on her a Kappa Tau Alpha journalism key for scholarship.

The Vasses have four daughters, all born in the Belgium Congo. Noteworthy among her many publications is the biography of her father, Dr. Eugene Kellersberger, Doctor Not Afraid. She is retired and resides in Dallas, Texas.

Chapter 4

Paraguay: Featuring John and Clara Schmidt (1946–1965)

by Edgar Stoesz

Other than the steady hum of powerful diesel engines and waves splashing against their huge ship, little was to be heard and even less was to be seen. Dr. John and Clara Schmidt and their five children were on the high seas on the mighty S.S. *Brazil,* somewhere between New York and Rio de Janeiro. Their destination? Paraguay, that little known, obscure, landlocked country, deep in the heart of South America where Mennonites had fled to escape Stalin's harsh persecution.

It was August 1951. World War II was over and Europe and Japan were rebuilding, but the world was not at peace. The cold war pervaded everything as testing was underway for yet more terrible weapons of destruction. A new conflict was brewing in South Asia.

This ten-day interlude gave the Schmidt couple an opportunity to reflect and anticipate. Both had grown up on farms in Kansas, the grandchildren of immigrants; John, Russian and Clara, Prussian. Both had received their elementary education in one-room country schools. They had experienced two World Wars and a Depression that left its mark on them. Both grew up in Mennonite churches where they came to faith in Jesus Christ, leading to a life of service. Who could have imagined how God would use this couple to bring healing and hope to leprosy sufferers in Paraguay and beyond?

Schmidt had what he described as a mediocre academic record in high school. Though tied down with farm chores, he managed to letter in basketball. Not sure what he wanted to do with his life, Schmidt followed his brother Herb to Kansas State University. Whereas Herb studied medicine, Schmidt was drawn to chemical engineering. Challenged by the demands of calculus, he decided to give medicine a try, something he had vowed not to do. One of two thousand applicants applying for seventy-seven positions, he rewarded his selection for medical school with a trip to the 1933 World's Fair in Chicago.

To his amazement, he liked medicine and did well in it, despite the demands of working to pay his way. For his internal medicine internship, he chose St. Joseph's Hospital in Baltimore. His three-year internship occurred while the nation was at war. Life more than a thousand miles away from home was lonely. He was drawn to the opposite sex, but vowed, "marriage or profession, not both."

The end of Schmidt's internship coincided with the Mennonite Central Committee (MCC) search for a physician to serve a community of two thousand people it had helped emigrate from Russia to Paraguay in 1930. These refugees had a heritage similar to the Schmidts's but, whereas the

Schmidt ancestors were part of a large migration to the American Midwest and Canada in the 1870s, the main Mennonite communities had remained in Russia, not knowing the fate awaiting them.

There followed in Russia what was called the Golden Era as Mennonites learned to farm the Russian steppes and created prosperous communities, making them the envy of their neighbors. All this came to a crashing halt when the cruel proletarian revolution swept through the countryside at the close of World War I. The harshest treatment was reserved for the Mennonites due to their comparative wealth and German loyalties. Their farms were taken away. Their churches and schools were closed. Family life was disrupted as many fathers were killed or deported to Siberia.

In 1924, the door opened for thousands to immigrate, mostly to Canada where they populated the frontier. Temporarily, things in Russia seemed more hopeful. Then, without warning, Joseph Stalin imposed new restrictions with a vengeance on those Mennonites who had remained. The threatened Mennonites feared that their decisions to stay had been a fatal error. Their cries to God and the Russian authorities for deliverance went unanswered.

Then suddenly and without explanation, five thousand were given permission to leave Moscow in 1929. They were dropped off in Germany, but were only promised temporary asylum there. Mennonite Central Committee, then a fledgling relief organization headquartered in Akron, Pennsylvania, joined in a desperate search for options. An offer from Brazil attracted some, though it was compromised in that it did not guarantee military exemption. Canada accepted only those that could meet its stringent health requirements. The United States did not open its doors, and joining them to the Old Colony Mennonites in Northern Mexico was not an acceptable plan. This left Paraguay as the only option.

Three years earlier, a community of two thousand Canadian Mennonites had pioneered a migration to Paraguay, establishing Menno Colony. Paraguay offered an unconditional welcome—young and old, sick and well, all were welcome. This generosity was motivated in part by the fact that some years earlier, Paraguay's male population had been decimated in a costly war with Brazil, Uruguay, and Argentina. Paraguay was additionally interested in populating the vast, isolated, sparsely populated Chaco region. Mennonites offered what Paraguay needed; it was a fit.

The new colony chose as its name Fernheim—home in the distance—secretly hoping to return to the farms they had fled from in Russia. Soon after their 1930 arrival in Paraguay, they found themselves engulfed in the Chaco war between Paraguay and Bolivia. Neither of the warring parties had paid much attention to the Chaco previously, not even bothering to establish clear boundaries. A rumor that oil was to be found there and the sudden influx of thousands of Mennonites changed all that. Mennonites found themselves "Innocent Pawns in the Chaco War," to quote the headline used by the *Christian Century* for an article in 1932. The war plus drought and pestilence, in addition to the unfriendly climate, made life unbelievably hard, but the Mennonites persisted, and eventually prospered.

Rain and medical help were on every list of needs. The search for a resident doctor proved to be as fruitless as calls for rain. Paraguayan doctors helped out occasionally, but fifteen years after their arrival, the two Mennonite communities, numbering more than four thousand people, remained a ten-day journey removed from medical care and almost everything else.

MCC's persistent search for a doctor led to Dr. Herbert Schmidt in Newton, Kansas. Herb Schmidt was unable to free himself from his thriving practice, but volunteered that his brother John, about to complete his internship in Baltimore, might be available. His telegram informing him of this unexpected development was waiting for John Schmidt when he returned from vacation. Turning to his friends, all frantically planning their next move, the soon-to-be-graduated doctor announced, "I'm going to Paraguay." They were shocked; most had never heard of the place.

His internship finished, Schmidt returned to his home in Kansas to say his good-byes. He had seen his family only once in three years. While making rounds with Herb, he chanced to notice a student nurse who would one day test his "marriage or profession" vow.

En route to Paraguay, Schmidt rendezvoused with Orie O. Miller at the Akron, Pennsylvania MCC headquarters. Miller was then MCC executive director and later to be chairman of the American Leprosy Missions. Passport, visa, and last-minute shopping and packing were completed in a flurry. On June 7, 1941, this veteran churchman and the rookie doctor boarded a ship in New York, headed for Rio de Janeiro. The eighteen-day voyage provided ample opportunity for Miller, an experienced traveler, to orient his thirty-year-old single recruit: term, one year; monthly salary, forty-five dollars plus room and board.

In Rio they transferred to a smaller ship for the onward journey to Asuncion. A still smaller ship awaited them in Asuncion for the trip up the Paraguay River to Puerto Casado, a company town regarded as the capital of the vast expanse and almost unpopulated territory known as the Chaco Boreal. After another two days' journey by train and ox cart through wilderness country into the interior, they arrived in Filadelfia, capital of Fernheim Colony. The narrow-gauge, Casado-owned train moved so slowly that when a sudden wind relieved Schmidt of his hat, he was able to retrieve it and reboard the train one car later.

Schmidt found a twelve-bed hospital with little more than the bare walls and a line of patients waiting to be seen. His trunk with clothing and supplies, however, was not received until his term was half over.

Much was strange in these new tropical surroundings, not the least of which was adjusting from the heat of the Kansas summer to the Paraguayan winter. The practice of medicine

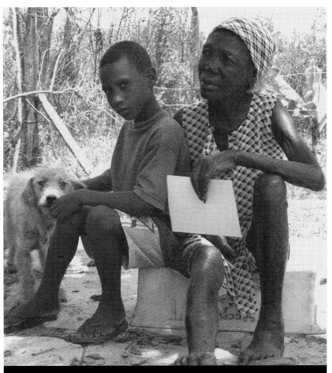

After India, Brazil has the most leprosy cases in the world. Carlos and his aunt receive care through an ALM program in Nova Iguacu.

called for ingenuity and innovation. It was not medicine as he had been taught. Distilled water was made with an improvised still. To treat anemia, the result of inadequate diet and the prevalence of parasites, rust was scraped from Chaco war machines and prepared as a medication. To lower the exceedingly high birth rate in the pre-pill era, the single doctor advised couples to sleep back-to-back. The basics of good health care were provided under these primitive conditions regardless: of the twelve cases of typhoid that occurred during his short stint, only one resulted in death.

But there was also familiarity. Schmidt was able to converse in Low German, the language his ancestors spoke in Russia. But he really felt at home when his Paraguayan host served him ammonia cookies, baked with the same recipe his grandmother brought with her from Russia seventy-five years earlier.

Mail was agonizingly slow and unreliable. Even so, he had several low-key exchanges with that student nurse he had met in Kansas.

With no replacement in sight when his one-year term was drawing to a close, Schmidt agreed to a six-month extension. In November 1941, it was with mixed feelings but much satisfaction that he left the Chaco, not expecting to return. With a suitcase in each hand, a souvenir pelt under each arm, and a big black hat on his head, he made his way overland to Chile where he boarded a ship for New Orleans via the Panama Canal and Cuba.

He arrived in Kansas City's Union Station late at night unshaven and disheveled from weeks of third-class travel. There to greet him was that student nurse, Clara Regier.

Adjusting back to life in the United States was made more difficult as World War II was in full swing. In 1942, Schmidt took a job in Albuquerque, New Mexico, but knew immediately that this was not to be his future home. Brother Herb's father-in-law, P. A. Penner, a veteran Mennonite missionary, invited Schmidt to join the India leprosy mission, but Schmidt had other things on his mind.

The relationship with Clara Regier quickly blossomed into a romance. She is described in the book *Garden in the Wilderness* as a nurse with a missionary spirit, crowned with a generous dose of adventure.

Five days after she received her RN degree in 1943, they were married. The young couple, full of hope and excitement, left the next day for a three-year term in Paraguay. When his bride asked what to pack, Schmidt replied, "We don't need much. The people have everything there." Their monthly pay? Seventy dollars plus room and board.

This time, travel was by airplane. But it was wartime and they were on a stand-by basis, making them subject to being bumped by military personnel. After numerous intermediate stops, they finally arrived in Asuncion. From there they made their way up the Paraguay River to the Chaco, as Schmidt had done a few years earlier. They continued by narrow-gauge, slow-moving company railroad

to the end station and on by ox cart, arriving in Filadelfia after dark. Schmidt had some idea what to expect, but Clara's curiosity would need to wait until morning.

Wagons rattling their way to the little Filadelfia hospital awakened them out of a deep sleep. People came in droves to welcome Schmidt back, to meet his new wife, and to present them with illnesses big and small. "I had to think of Jesus going around healing," opined Mrs. Schmidt, obviously proud of her new husband.

Schmidt was in his element, but for his wife it was total emersion. Her tasks were many as receptionist, surgical assistant, and nursing instructor, in addition to wife and soon-to-be mother. In the evening she taught piano and typing, and helped her husband with Bible studies. Sometimes the tensions of surgery overtaxed their equipment and training, creating tensions they took home with them to the same one-room apartment Schmidt occupied when he was single.

A schoolteacher was trained to serve as an anesthetist. A former woodworker became the pharmacist. Young women, intelligent and motivated but with limited education, were taught to serve as nurse's aides. Educational materials the couple brought with them from home were translated from English into German.

The Schmidts's first born, John Russell, was born on the coldest night of the year. His father proudly signed the birth certificate, "Doctor, Father and Nurse." Eighteen months later, Elizabeth was welcomed in the heat of summer.

Satisfying and rewarding as it was, Clara Schmidt had envisioned mission work differently. She was not convinced that this was for what she had dedicated her life. Chaco Mennonites seemed so focused on getting established in this foreign and hostile environment that most showed little interest in their Indian and Paraguayan neighbors. The isolation felt stifling.

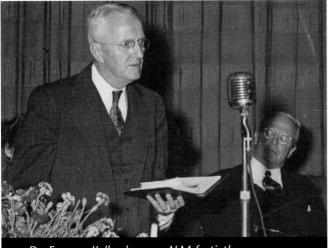
Dr. Eugene Kellersberger, ALM fortieth anniversary, 1946

As their term was drawing to a close, they became aware through Disciples of Christ missionaries that leprosy existed in Paraguay, with estimates as high as thirty thousand cases. (Later this estimate was lowered to six thousand.) E. R. Kellersberger, then president of the American Leprosy Missions, was so moved by what he found on a survey trip that he pledged fifty thousand dollars to start a new service.

The Schmidts were also aware that thought was being given to an appropriate way for Mennonites to thank Paraguay for welcoming them when no other nation would have them. Though life in Paraguay had been hard, and their future still uncertain, they were now free and still hopeful. The question was what form this expression of gratitude should take.

No one remembers exactly who suggested it first, but somehow the two ideas were joined. How better to thank Paraguay than by undertaking a project to care for the neediest in their midst? They could not have known all that would cost them in money and effort, nor the satisfaction it would bring them.

Schmidt was among the first to seize on the idea. Shortly before their departure for the United States, Schmidt joined a delegation of Mennonite leaders to make the first exploratory trip. Their term ended in September 1946 and they returned to Kansas

with two children, feeling their work in Paraguay was finished.

After a brief interlude in Freeman, South Dakota, their wish to practice medicine and raise their family in a Mennonite community appeared realized with an invitation from Mountain Lake, Minnesota. Everything seemed set for the next phase of their lives with one major obstacle. Schmidt had a serious ulcer problem, dating back to his medical school days, now exacerbated by the pressures of starting a new practice in a new community. He was living on pudding and baby food. This was corrected when doctors at the Mayo Clinic surgically removed four-fifths of his stomach.

Happy and fulfilled as they were, Schmidt observed "we couldn't get Paraguay out of our minds." Especially irrepressible was the memory of victims of leprosy and an appropriate way to say thank you to Paraguay. Their curiosity got the better of them. They asked MCC for a progress report. Some years later Clara Schmidt exclaimed, "We really stuck our foot into it!" MCC invited them to become the first directors of the project still in the planning stage.

In the meanwhile, planning in Paraguay lurched forward amid many obstacles. Mennonite leaders, like the Schmidts, were unable to let go of the vision. Where? Who? How? What seemed promising in one meeting was cancelled before the next. In the middle of it all Paraguay had another of the political revolutions for which it was famous, bringing everything to a halt.

Before agreeing to disrupt their comfortable lives, Schmidt insisted on visiting the only United States-based leprosy center, located in Carville, Louisiana. Here he learned about the sulphone drugs that offered the long-awaited cure and the discovery that leprosy was not as contagious as once thought. Perhaps new forms of treatment could be considered. In discussions that lasted far into the night, Schmidt and Carville doctors concluded that home treatment was worth a try. Perhaps soon putting "lepers" away in isolated colonies could be regarded as a thing of the past.

Schmidt's health restored, the couple accepted the MCC invitation on two conditions: that the program be owned and directed by Mennonites in Paraguay, and that it be supported by Mennonite Central Committee and the American Leprosy Missions. Decision on treatment methodology was deferred. Now the Schmidt family, with five children and seventy-four crates of supplies, was on its way to Paraguay, full of hope, but also with some well-founded anxiety.

Upon arrival in 1964, they discovered that planning was less advanced than anticipated. Following the custom of the day, Paraguay maintained a leprosy colony at Sapucai, near the remote town of Santa Isabel. Here victims were destined to live out their days, removed from public view and interaction. The project Mennonites had in mind was an upgrade of that model. The government of Paraguay offered a twenty-thousand-hectare tract of land near Conception. It met the first requirement—isolation.

Upon closer inspection it was found that ninety-two squatter families had put prior claim to parts of the designated tract. The mayor offered to have the military evict them, but the Mennonite committee found that totally unacceptable. Everything was once again at a standstill. In reflecting on all their reverses and frustrations, some began to ask, "If this is God's will, why is it so difficult?"

The search for an alternate location led to a 1,148-hectare (2,835-acre) tract of gently rolling land near Itacuribi, eighty-one kilometers from Asuncion, giving it the nickname Km. 81 by which it is known to this day. Located on the road leading to Brazil and the world-famous Iguazu Falls, it happened also to be an area with high leprosy prevalence. With the exception of two dilapidated buildings, it was bare land. But would the community welcome a leprosy service?

The answer was not long in coming. One Sunday afternoon, after the foundations were in place for what was to be the Schmidt house, neighbors came to protest, well fortified with rocks. Schmidt was in Brazil, supplementing the leprosy gap in his medical training, but his wife explained in limited Spanish that this was intended to be their residence. Sensing that she was not being understood, she served the angry men coffee and cookies. They left some hours later, taking with them the rocks they had brought to reinforce their point. A soft answer had turned away wrath!

Later it was learned that the community people were so fearful of being tainted by a leprosy colony that they lodged a protest with Paraguay's President Alfredo Stroessner. Stroessner, favorable to Mennonites throughout his long reign, dismissed it by saying, "I wish the Mennonites would build a leprosy hospital in every corner of Paraguay."

While the venue had changed, thoughts about treatment methodology continued along traditional lines—a leper *colony*. Convincing the Paraguay Mennonite Committee, Mennonite Central Committee, and even the American Leprosy Missions and the government of Paraguay to pioneer a new treatment method was daunting. Things reached such an impasse that MCC and ALM threatened to withdraw their funding, causing the Schmidts to wonder if they would need to terminate.

In the heat of the debate Dr. Federico Rio, former director of the Santa Isabel Colony, weighed in with a timely, thirteen-page letter giving a ringing endorsement to the ambulatory treatment approach.

To assuage resistance from the local community, and to respond to medical needs of the surrounding area, a general clinic was initiated along with the leprosy service. But few leprosy patients came. Three years after the Schmidts's 1951 arrival in Paraguay, they had treated just fourteen leprosy patients. In a speech laced with emotion, Schmidt said to his impatient critics, "They (leprosy patients) are out there. We must go find them."

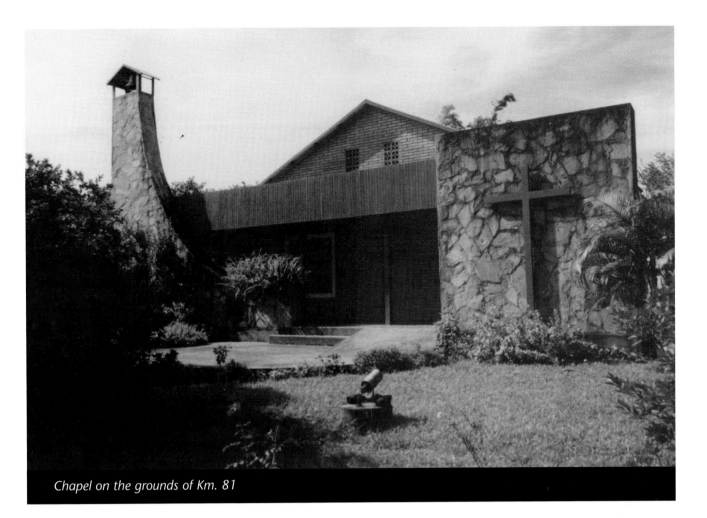

Chapel on the grounds of Km. 81

Case-finding teams were organized into search missions. With a four-wheel-drive army Jeep, or more often on horseback, they scoured the countryside, often traveling at night to escape the heat, sometimes sleeping in the open or on church benches.

Social stigma was the culprit. Fearing deportation to the dreaded colony, persons with signs of leprosy either hid or were ostracized by well-intended but frightened families. Search teams learned that "the more vehement the denial that someone with leprosy was in their midst, the closer we are to finding another patient." Some victims absented themselves voluntarily to spare their families embarrassment, accepting the life of a vagrant.

Frustration that leprosy patients did not respond to routine medical treatment and the belief that leprosy was a curse from God drove more than one well-intending family to forcibly hold a victim over fire, hoping in this way to cleanse him from this disfiguring curse.

The Program Gains Acceptance

Gradually, persistence and a growing reputation brought about increased public acceptance. From 1953 to July 1955, the Km. 81 register recorded 516 patients. The number treated was far in excess of what would have been possible using the outdated colony method. The local community came to accept this uninvited treatment center and the Paraguayan Health Ministry became supportive of the ambulatory form of home treatment.

Staff for the growing program came mostly from the three Mennonite colonies in the Chaco

Antonia and Nicholas Missena

First, mother Antonia, and then her twelve-year-old son Nicholas were found to have leprosy. They knew the fate that awaited them in the pre-cure era. Nicholas watched as his mother went to each of her sleeping children and took a tearful, predawn leave of them. Soldiers escorted them to the train that would take them to the Santa Isabel Leper Colony. First was the locomotive, then the passenger cars, then the freight car reserved for them! The heat was as unbearable as the humiliation and uncertainty.

Arriving at the station, they heard yelling. "Leproso! Leproso! Leproso!" Then the wagon was given a thorough washing.

Maintaining a safe distance, soldiers ordered mother and son to march to the leper colony some miles distant. When they came to a place where children were playing, the children suddenly scattered. Had a mad dog suddenly appeared, or what was the explanation? Nicholas asked the soldier to explain. "The children are afraid of you," he replied gruffly. The memory of this humiliation stayed with Nicholas for the rest of his life.

After some hours in the hot sun, Antonia was fatigued and desperately thirsty, but no rest stop was permitted. Exhausted, she sagged into the tall grass at the side of the road. Mother and son were able eventually to resume their march and arrived at the leper colony late in the day. The soldier turned them over to be enrolled. After *maté* and *gallettas* (Paraguayan drink and biscuit) they toured what was to be their new home. Nicholas looked in vain for children with whom he could play football and for the hospital where his leprosy would be treated.

Now fifteen years of age, Nicholas was totally absorbed with himself and his future. Every day he sat looking at his disfigured face in a mirror, longing for the beautiful complexion of normal children. In disgust he crashed the mirror to the dirt floor and resigned himself to seek help from Dona Brigida, known as the "burn healer." She greeted Nicholas in a friendly manner. Sensing his apprehension, she told him about her successes and assured him that his young face would heal quickly and be as smooth and beautiful as the pictures he admired.

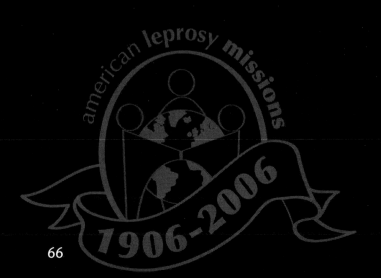

With growing apprehension, Nicholas entered the shabby hut, noticing holes in the roof. Dona Brigida proceeded to stoke a hot fire to sterilize her instruments. As the fire got hotter and the instruments turned cherry red, Nicholas's courage sank. *This women must be a sadist to torture people with such treatment.* He felt like a lamb about to be slaughtered, but then reminded himself how good it would feel to have a beautiful face like other children.

Seeing the irons in the fire and imagining them applied to his face, he had an urge to urinate and so asked to be excused. Dona Brigida had assumed a position that gave her complete control over Nicholas's movements. She refused his request, saying the procedure was about to begin. With her right hand she took a firm grip on his forehead while with the left hand she forced the red-hot iron against his face. The pain was excruciating. He was nauseated by the smell and the crackling sound of burning flesh.

Her grip grew tighter as the treatment was repeated, one red-hot iron after another. Finally, unable to resist or scream, Nicholas resigned himself in exhaustion. The embarrassment of soiled pants was the least of his worries.

Dona Brigida in the meanwhile assured him that the procedure had gone well and that she had gotten to the root of his problems. Soon, she assured him, he would have a pretty face—"like normal children."

The ensuing night was unforgettably long and painful. In his delirium Nicholas visualized thousands of lepra bacilli imprisoned in his body, resisting expulsion. The next morning Antonia was horrified at the sight of Nicholas. He assured her that all would be well when the swelling subsided. But it was not. The treatment only made his skin worse.

Nicholas and his mother continued to live at Santa Isabel for some years. Nicholas eventually married a fellow colony resident, not knowing that this was forbidden. Both responded well to a new drug treatment and were permitted to leave the colony. They found their way to Km. 81 where ALM-trained Dr. Duerksen performed several surgeries to restore Nicholas's disfigured face.

—condensed and translated by Edgar Stoesz
from *Hospital Mennonita Km 81: Liebe, die taetig wird*
by Gerhard Ratzlaff

Nety Voth

Nety Voth was a resident of Friesland, a Mennonite colony in East Paraguay. She ventured to Filadelfia in 1944 at age eighteen to complete a nurse-training course offered by Clara Schmidt. Her coworkers watched helplessly as she slipped into a diabetic coma, her supply of insulin having been exhausted. Her life was in the balance when radio contact was made with the MCC office in Asuncion. With help from the American Embassy, a supply of insulin was located and dispatched to the Chaco by airplane. There being no airstrip in the Chaco, the insulin was dropped with an improvised parachute. It landed near the hospital in the nick of time. Voth's life was spared. When the Km. 81 program opened in 1951, she became its first nurse. Nety Voth rendered loving service until her death at age thirty-nine, whereupon she was buried at Km. 81.

—condensed and translated
by Edgar Stoesz
from *Hospital Mennonita Km 81:
Liebe, die taetig wird* by Gerhard Ratzlaff

Idole Boese

Idole Boese, after being diagnosed with leprosy, was handcuffed and marched several days by armed soldiers to the state run colony in Santa Isabel. Here he was left to live out his days. It was his good fortune to be discovered by a Km. 81 search team, cured and later employed.

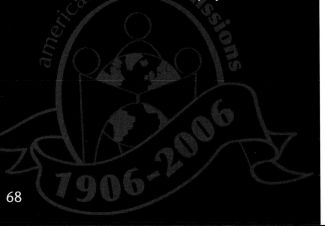

located some four hundred kilometers distant, and from the Mennonite colonies of Friesland and Volendam in East Paraguay. Notable among staff are Hans Penner and Gerhard Pries, who together logged fifteen years in case-finding missions, and Hans Regehr who served as chaplain.

"John Schmidt . . . was the first to try such a venture, and it has become the basis for leprosy-control work throughout the world today. It has virtually eliminated the need for 'settlements' of several decades ago," said Dr. Oliver Hasselblad, president of the American Leprosy Missions in 1967. Instead of earning the dubious distinction of being one of the last to build a leper colony, Paraguay became a pioneer in this new form of ambulatory treatment.

Though predicated on the ambulatory home treatment model, a support base was needed for surgery and other support services, including housing for a growing staff and homeless patients. One building was added after another until it became a mini village. Always, it seemed, something was under construction.

Laid out before the decision was made to go the ambulatory route, the residential and treatment zones were separated by a three-hundred-meter corridor (reduced from the three previously thought necessary). Schmidt later referred to this separation as the "*avenida de ignorancia*" (the avenue of ignorance).

A Comprehensive Treatment Approach

Km. 81 was from the outset a ministry to the whole person—body, mind, and soul. The motto was, and remains, "In the Service of Love." Bible study and evangelism were part of the package. A chapel was built to provide a place of worship on the grounds. The first baptismal class in 1959 was comprised of seven patients. Many patients returned to their communities not only cured but also with a newfound faith. More than one former patient has been heard to praise God for having been inflicted by this dreaded disease, since in the process he or she was led to faith in Jesus Christ.

Ever the innovator, Schmidt introduced physiotherapy in 1966. A Canadian nurse, Eleanor Mathies, was recruited by MCC and, after some months of training in India, helped many regain limited use of hands and feet; she also trained other paraprofessional physiotherapists.

Next was the introduction of custom-made footwear. Though cured of the disease, many patients were left with badly deformed feet. With their ability to feel pain destroyed by leprosy, they were in danger of re-injuring themselves with footwear that did not conform to crippled feet. A Chaco Mennonite cobbler was enticed to relocate to Km. 81 in 1974. This service permitted patients to work in their gardens and live a near normal life. Today the cobbler shop makes shoes and prostheses for leprosy and non-leprosy patients for all of Paraguay.

A By-Product

Though the focus of Km. 81 was on leprosy, there was a second and, some would say an equally poignant dimension. While serving in the Chaco, Schmidt observed that Mennonite families were large and burdened by what he perceived as an isolation mentality. "They need a bigger view of the world."

Schmidt's Km. 81 paradigm wed these two dimensions. The program was predicated on a stream of short-term volunteers from the Mennonite colonies, modeled after the voluntary service program Schmidt had observed in Canada and the United States following World War II conscription. The seed took root as young people responded to the challenge. Some years later, Mennonite ministers observed: "When service workers return from a year at Km. 81 they bring a new vitality with them."

In year 2001, literally thousands of Mennonites came from all over Paraguay to a double golden celebration—fifty years of treating leprosy and fifty years of voluntary service. It was estimated that twelve hundred Mennonite volunteers had served at Km. 81 a year or more, and many more in other social services including the state psychiatric hospital in Asuncion.

The grounds were beautifully manicured for the celebration. Speakers, including ALM president Christopher Doyle, expressed satisfaction over how this modest beginning had been blessed and used of God for the benefit of many. The benefits had clearly been reciprocal.

The Schmidt Era Ends

Having navigated it through the first crucial twenty years, the Schmidts turned the Km. 81 program over to Dr. Frank Duerksen and his helpmate wife, Anne, in 1971, when Schmidt was sixty years of age. Children of Mennonite immigrants, Duerksen received his medical training in Argentina where he met Anne. With the help of ALM, he studied specialized hand surgery with Dr. Paul Brand in Ethiopia. When their Paraguay term of service was finished, the Duerksen family relocated to Winnipeg, Manitoba, Canada, but he continued annual trips of weeks', or even months', duration to teach and advise leprosy programs in Brazil and Paraguay. The fruit of his labors abounds.

A succession of Mennonite doctors followed, but the original vision has remained constant. From 1994 to 2003 the program was under the direction of Dr. Carlos Wiens and his nurse wife, Carla, both grandchildren of Chaco immigrants. Wiens was born at Km. 81, attended by Schmidt when his parents served there as chaplains. He grew up playing with neighborhood children, giving him command of Spanish and local Indian languages, in addition to the German and Low German still spoken by many Mennonites. Wiens graduated first in his medical class, giving him his choice of positions available. To the surprise of most and the disappointment of some, this promising doctor chose to dedicate himself to the treatment of leprosy.

After almost ten years of meritorious service as medical director, Dr. Wiens assumed the position of director general of health of Paraguay.

In twenty years, the bare, gently rolling hillsides have been converted into a village of refuge—a village with houses, trees, and acres of manicured lawns and flowerbeds, with a hospital/clinic/chapel at its center, swarming with people, some on crutches, many with bandages—an oasis of sorts for the healing of body and soul. The program has been expanded beyond leprosy and serves the medical needs of the general population, although leprosy remains its primary focus. Search teams continue to scour the countryside for new victims of a disease that can now be cured but not yet prevented.

A Legacy Continues

John, always with Clara at his side, continued in a variety of voluntary services—some medical, some very routine, sometimes in Paraguay, sometimes in Kansas or Vietnam. He died in Filadelfia, Paraguay, on November 6, 2003 at the age of ninety-two. He was recognized at his funeral as a pioneer, a man of vision, driven by a desire to honor God and

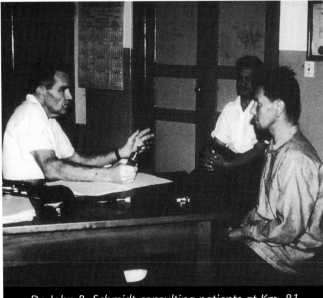

Dr. John R. Schmidt consulting patients at Km. 81

serve others. Clara continues to reside in the Mennonite retirement home in Filadelfia.

The Schmidt children grew up and made their way into the world. Three sons— a rancher, a doctor, and a missionary—and two foster children and their families reside in Paraguay. Three daughters live in the United States.

A Partnership Model

Although Paraguay Mennonites took the lead, Km. 81 was and remains the work of multiple partners, spanning more than fifty years.

- The Government of Paraguay sanctioned the program and expanded the assigned territory until today it covers all of Paraguay, and offers valuable collaboration to neighboring countries.

- The Mennonite colonies in the Chaco and East Paraguay have used it as their way of saying thank you to Paraguay for opening its doors to them. Having generously supported it with personnel and money, they rightfully claim it as their own.

- The workers, hundreds, even thousands have served faithfully, some years, others only months, but all have left their contribution.

- The Mennonite Central Committee supported the effort from its conception through Orie O. Miller serving in a dual role as executive director of MCC and chairman of ALM. MCC found the Schmidts and other workers, and supplemented the budget.

- American Leprosy Missions contributed valuable professional expertise and substantial funding, supplemented also by other ILEP members.

Halfway Around the World—Almost!

In 1960 John and Clara Schmidt with their six children, ages ranging from three to sixteen, boarded their retrofitted Volvo, christened "Old Faithful," in Asuncion, Paraguay, and headed due North. Destination: Newton, Kansas—some more than 11,000 miles distant.

Sometimes the roads were so challenging, everyone but the chauffeur got out to push. Other times there was no road, or a road without bridges.

Fresh fruit and bread and other staples like rice and potatoes were bought along the way. Lodging was found with missionaries en route or, in dire circumstances, in vacant church buildings.

Two nights and one day were spent on a freighter making the connection between Columbia and Panama. While in Panama, they rendezvoused with Dr. Arthur Klassen, the most recent MCC recruit en route to Paraguay to do replacement duty.

In Nicaragua an accommodating immigration official handed the Schmidts a letter written by a missionary who heard about their trip on radio HCJB Quito and invited them to spend the night with her. So unique was this traveling troupe that the official had no difficulty recognizing them.

Schmidt did most of the driving, assisted by sixteen-year-old J. R. Clara wrote the trip diary and kept order in the car. The children whiled away the time by working on their correspondence courses, knitting, and playing cabin games. Each day began with the family singing "Father we thank thee for the night."

Ninety-four-and-one-half long, tedious days later, on May 22, they completed their 11,187-mile journey with much rejoicing, having had no serious illness, no accident, and just one flat tire. The experience and the friendships made along the way remained a lifelong memory.

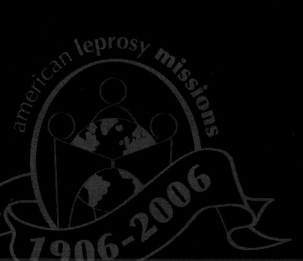

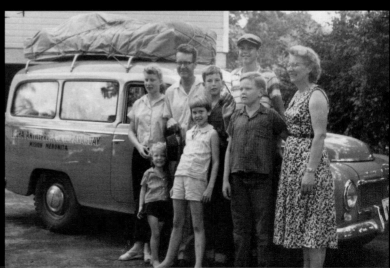

Dona Maria

Maria Haseitl was born into a large, poor family. Instead of going to school, she had to work to supplement the family income. In her teens, she had the fortune of meeting and falling in love with Adolph. Soon they were blessed with a son. Through hard work they were able to acquire a small farm. In her words they were "unbelievably happy."

One day Adolph saw a blister on Maria's arm and asked if she had burned herself. She was unaware of the blister, having lost feeling. Leprosy was suspected, but test results were negative.

Additional tests also came back negative, but as a precaution the doctor ordered her to be isolated. A little house was built for her and, though she had the basics, it was hard to live apart from her family. One of the few activities left for her was to gather firewood and help with making charcoal. The worry, isolation, and loneliness were nearly unbearable.

Desperate for help, they consulted a specialist. After a thorough examination they heard the dreaded diagnosis—leprosy. Maria was ordered to the leper colony in Santa Isabel. She gathered up some clothes, a blanket her mother had given her as a wedding present, and a few cooking utensils and, with a heavy heart, she and Adolph left on the four-day trip.

Upon arrival, fatigue and apprehension gave way to revulsion. They were shown to the women's quarters, housed in a dilapidated building that resembled a barn. Quickly they were encircled—everybody wanted to see the new resident. Some without fingers, others without toes, some with neither. Some had no eyebrows. One had no nose! What a welcoming party!

Maria was in tears. And poor Adolph: How could he leave the wife he loved in such a place? It was both frustrating and a relief when the chauffeur insisted it was time to leave. Their farewell, she said, was "indescribable." Maria watched as the car disappeared. Then she cried until she could cry no more. It would be eighteen years before she would see her husband again.

Maria lived in this state of shock for months—maybe years—with only the occasional reprieve. Then one day someone extended a hand to her and asked, "And how are you, Dona Maria?" She was shocked. Looking to see who was addressing her in a respectful manner, she found herself looking into the smiling face of a Salvation Army preacher. "I am very unhappy," was her answer. He replied, "Seek Jesus."

She was troubled by this exchange. It nevertheless caused her to do some thinking. She dug out the Bible and read it, but nothing spoke to her. Then she was drawn into a Bible study that eventually led her to experience peace in Christ.

Eventually Maria adjusted, and on occasions, even experienced some humor. Snakes visited their humble surroundings frequently but, as someone observed, no one was ever bitten. Why? A variety of reasons were offered but the resounding conclusion was that even snakes detested their smell and shunned them!

One day Maria fell, resulting in an injury that could only be corrected by surgery. Surgery was beyond her means. Would she be required to live out her days with this additional affliction? She appealed to Adolph and son Edwin. Her letter traced them to the Hutterite colony, Primavera, in East Paraguay where they had gone to find work. When the Hutterite congregation learned of her need, they dispatched a plane to get her so her surgery could be performed in their hospital.

After surgery her leprosy was cured with medication and she was reunited with her family. Maria could hardly believe her sudden change in fortune. The family eventually moved to Uruguay and from there to the Hutterite Bruderhof in Connecticut, where Adolph died in 1985. Maria died in 1988 at the age of eighty-eight.

**—condensed and translated
by Edgar Stoesz
from Hospital Mennonita Km 81:
Liebe, die taetig wird by Gerhard Ratzlaff**

Gertrude Unruh

Gertrude Unruh was chief nurse at Km. 81 when she developed abdominal problems. Dr. Schmidt recommended that she be seen by Dr. Dowell, a missionary doctor colleague at the Asuncion Baptist Hospital. Dowell diagnosed inoperable ovarian cancer and released her to return to Km. 81 to live out her days. Unruh quietly resigned herself to continue serving as long as possible.

Many years later, when Dr. Wesley Schmidt, son of John and Clara, was a physician at Km. 81, he was surprised to find Unruh still serving as the chief nurse. "She taught me more in her quiet way than any of my Paraguayan and American professors ever had," Wesley Schmidt said.

Gertrude Unruh eventually retired to Filadelfia. Thirty years after the first cancer appeared, she came to Wesley, then a physician at the Asuncion Baptist Hospital, complaining about abdominal pain. It was Wesley's place to inform this "elderly angel" that she really had an inoperable cancer. They shared some tears of gratitude to the Lord for the gift of the thirty years to serve others. A few weeks later she went peacefully to be with her Lord.

—Wesley Schmidt

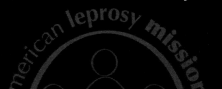

we went to find them," he said. After two years he returned to his home in Friesland Colony exhausted, but he could not forget those suffering with leprosy. When invited in 1959 to continue under a parallel program with the Paraguayan Ministerium, he gladly accepted.

To reach those most inaccessible more quickly, he furnished his own horse, sometimes with wagon. Monday through Saturday (home for Sunday, if possible), he pursued leads for new contacts, followed up on delinquent patients, and delivered medicines. Finding that people accepted him more readily when he addressed them in Guarani, he worked to enlarge his vocabulary. Families he served provided night lodging and meals. This led to such unique experiences as being awakened by a pig scratching itself on his bedpost.

What Arndt Funk lacked in formal training, he more than made up for in native ability. He was able to identify the lepra bacillis under the microscope and he understood the medications. Most valuable of all, he had a heart of Christian compassion, a supportive family, and a durable body.

Now retired in a rest home in Friesland Colony, he said in his native German, "Our generation will not have the last word with leprosy." Looking back over a career that spanned thirty-six years, he left no doubt that he felt totally fulfilled

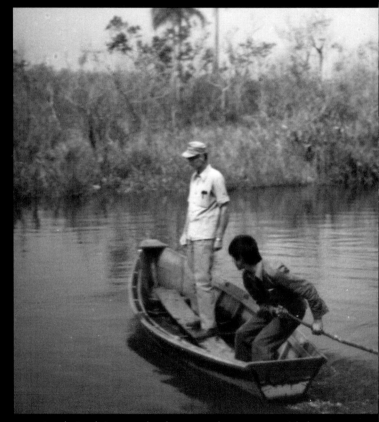

Arndt Funk in search of yet another person with leprosy

ABOUT THE AUTHOR

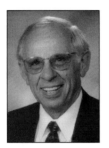

*E*dgar Stoesz grew up in Mountain Lake, Minnesota. After attending the University of Minnesota, he married and elected to do alternative service with the Mennonite Central Committee (MCC). He retired from thirty-four years with MCC, having served in six administrative roles, including director of international programs.

Stoesz has served on numerous boards including twelve years on American Leprosy Missions, three years as chair; seven years on Habitat For Humanity International, four years as chair; eight years on the board of Heifer Project International, two years as chair; eight years on the Executive Committee of Mennonite Economic Development Associates; and numerous others.

He has authored numerous articles and six books, including Garden in the Wilderness: Mennonite Communities in the Paraguayan Chaco and Doing Good Better, *a guide for nonprofit boards, now also available in video form.*

Stoesz has traveled widely, visiting leprosy work on four continents. He resides with his wife, Gladys, in Akron, Pennsylvania. They have four grown children and seven grandchildren.

Chapter 5

India: Featuring Paul and Margaret Brand (1966–1985)

by Philip Yancey

Two young British students met in medical school, married in 1943, and served out their residency years during World War II as German bombers produced massive numbers of casualties all over England. Paul specialized in orthopedic surgery while Margaret pursued pediatrics.

Paul Brand's surgical residency ended in 1946, a year after World War II, at which time he fully expected to be shipped overseas with British occupation troops for a few years. Afterwards he planned to return to a quiet career in a research laboratory back in England. But the Central Medical War Committee, which oversaw such assignments, proved no match for an irrepressible Scotsman named Dr. Robert Cochrane.

The supervisor of leprosy work in southern India, Cochrane had come to London to recruit a surgeon for a new medical college in the town of Vellore. Somehow Cochrane persuaded the war committee to accept Brand's service in India in lieu of a mandatory army stint. For Brand, India represented home. The son of missionary parents there, he had often enchanted his bride with stories of growing up in the mountains among common village folk.

Brand embarked for India alone in order to fill the urgent need at Vellore and to allow his wife time to recover from the birth of their second child. Within a few days he was feeling Indian again. He went around barefoot or in sandals, and wore loose-fitting cotton clothes. He went to sleep beneath a slowly turning ceiling fan, soothed by the clear metallic "hoo . . . hoo" of the coppersmith birds, and awoke to the raucous sound of crows.

After six months, Margaret Brand and two small children set sail from England, and in June of 1947, the Brand family was reunited at last. They moved into the top floor of a stone bungalow near the medical college. Margaret Brand joined her husband at the hospital, where she had taken a position in pediatrics.

The Vellore hospital had been founded in 1900 by an American missionary, Dr. Ida Scudder. It began as a medical college for young women, based initially in a small dispensary that measured no more than ten feet by twelve feet. The school flourished, and eventually opened its doors to male students. By the time the Brands arrived, the Vellore hospital had grown into a sprawling four-hundred-bed complex of buildings. Somehow, despite the hospital's size, the staff had retained the strong sense of Christian community that Dr. Scudder had first inspired.

Practicing medicine in India called for creativity. Something was always going wrong that no textbook had prepared them for: a power blackout in the middle of surgery, a report of rabies in the hospital, a water shortage, an unknown pyrogen in the blood bank. The doctors had to improvise on the spot.

A Faithful Assistant Rewarded

Young boys sometimes volunteered to assist at the eye camps, and Margaret was once assigned a shy, dark boy about twelve years old. He stood on a box, with an impressive but baggy hospital gown wrapped around him, charged with strict instructions to hold a three-battery flashlight—the village had no electricity—so that the light beamed directly on the cornea of the patient's eye. Margaret was dubious: Could a young village boy who had never watched any surgery endure the trauma of seeing people's eyes sliced open and stitched together again?

The child, however, performed his task with remarkable aplomb. During the first five operations he scrupulously followed Margaret's instructions on when to shift the angle of light, aiming the beam with a steady, confident hand. But during the sixth case he faltered. Margaret kept saying softly, "Little brother, show the light properly," which he would momentarily do, but soon it would again jerk dangerously away from where she was cutting.

Margaret could see that her assistant simply could not bear to look at the eye being worked on. She stopped and asked if he was feeling well. Tears ran down his cheeks and he stuttered, "Oh, doctor—I-I cannot look. This one, she is my mother."

Ten days later the boy's mother's stitches were removed, and the team gave her eyeglasses. She first tried to blink away the dazzling light, but finally adjusted, focused, and for the first time in her life saw her son. A smile creased her face as she reached out to touch him. "My son," she said, "I thought I knew you, but today I see you." And she pulled him close.

Medical Detours

Medical training during wartime had emphasized specialization and, as a result, students missed out on the full experience of rotations in all fields. Working on a short-term assignment in a mission station clinic, Margaret Brand felt her inadequacies most keenly in the field of ophthalmology. She watched with marvel as an American missionary diagnosed and treated the many eye afflictions common in India, sometimes preventing blindness, sometimes even restoring sight.

A year later, shortly before delivering her third child, the Vellore hospital asked Brand which department she would like to join. "Really, I don't care," she replied, "as long as it isn't in eyes." But the greatest need at Vellore in those days happened to be in the eye department. One day a bicycle courier delivered this message from the acting director: "Dear Margaret. We don't wish to hurry you, but we must have more help in the Eye Department as soon as possible. Carol."

Brand turned the piece of paper over and wrote: "Dear Carol, I don't mind being hurried but I know nothing about eyes. You'll have to look for someone else. Sorry. Margaret." She assumed that was the end.

But one hour later the messenger returned with another note that simply said: "You'll learn. Please start on Monday. Carol."

And learn she did. She happened to begin work at the height of an epidemic of keratoconjunctivitis, an infectious inflammation of the eye. That first morning, nearly four hundred patients were waiting in the clinic. Soon Brand was supervising an out-patient clinic swarming with patients suffering from infections and other eye disorders.

She also began accompanying a surgeon, Dr. Victor Rambo, on village visits. Cataracts had blinded thousands of people, including many children, and many of them could be restored to sight through a relatively simple surgical

Stigma and Science

The early history of leprosy tells of a saintly few who, defying society's stigma, looked past the unsightly symptoms of leprosy and ministered to its victims. As the disease ravaged Europe during the Middle Ages, orders of nuns devoted to Lazarus, the patron saint of leprosy, established homes for patients. These courageous women could do little but bind wounds and change dressings, but the homes themselves, called lazarettos, may have helped break the hold of the disease in Europe by isolating leprosy patients and improving their living conditions. In the nineteenth and twentieth centuries, Christian missionaries who spread across the globe established many colonies for leprosy patients, such as the one at Chingleput, and as a result many of the major scientific advances in understanding and treating leprosy came from missionaries—Bob Cochrane being the latest in a long line.

At Chingleput, the introduction of sulfone drugs represented an exciting breakthrough. The previous treatment, injecting oil distilled from the chaulmoogra tree directly into the patients' skin patches, had side effects almost as bad as the disease. Some doctors preferred many small injections, as many as 320 per week, which left the skin pulpy and inflamed for a time. Desperate, patients sought out such treatment, and some reported improvement. The new sulfone drug had the distinct advantage that it could be taken orally. And after five years of testing with sulfone, patients were actually showing negative reports of active bacteria. Leprosy had virtually disappeared from their bodies.

No longer contagious, their disease now inactive, these people could theoretically be released back to their villages. Hopes dimmed, however, as it became clear that villages had no interest in welcoming home anyone with a history of leprosy. In almost every case, patients chose to stay on at Chingleput even after they had been cured.

procedure. Rambo patiently taught Margaret techniques of cataract surgery, which she practiced on the eyes of animals obtained from the butcher. Rambo had established a regular regimen of "eye camps." Because many of the neediest people could not travel to the hospital, he and a team of helpers took a well-stocked mobile unit on monthly circuits into rural areas. On a certain date announced in advance, a designated building, perhaps a school or an old rice mill, would receive a stream of Indians afflicted with runny eyes or blindness. If no building was available, the Vellore team would set up portable operating tables under a banyan tree.

The entire team was comprised of doctors, nurses, medical students, skilled and non-skilled assistants, translators, evangelists, and cooks. They worked under crude conditions, sometimes in stifling heat, devising an assembly line of treatment. They even supplied musicians, as patients who had to lie quietly day after day following eye surgery needed some entertainment.

Some of the team would return to Vellore while others stayed for several days to care for the patients who had surgery. On follow-up visits, doctors removed stitches, treated infections, and fitted the proper eyewear. For their services the team charged each patient one rupee (approximately five cents). Margaret Brand had never worked so hard; on the eye camps, sometimes two doctors performed over one hundred cataract operations a day.

The Dangers of Losing Touch

In the weaving shop at Chingleput, Paul noticed one young boy working vigorously at a loom, shooting the shuttle through the weft with his right hand and then reaching out with his left hand to ram a wooden bar against the threads, forcing them together. He picked up speed, probably showing off for the director and his guest, and bits of cotton floated through the air like dust.

Paul noticed a trail of dark spots on the cotton cloth. Blood? "May I see your hand?" Paul yelled to the weaver. The boy released the pedals and set down the shuttle, and instantly the noise level in the room dropped several decibels. The weaver held out a deformed, twisted hand with shortened fingers. His index finger had lost maybe a third of an inch in length, and as Paul looked closer he saw naked bone protruding from a nasty, septic wound. This boy was working with a finger cut to the bone!

"How did you cut yourself?" Paul asked. He gave a nonchalant reply, "Oh, it's nothing. I had a pimple on my finger, and earlier it bled a little. I guess it's opened up again." Paul took a few photos of his hand to add to his orthopedics files, and the doctors dispatched him to the clinic for bandaging.

"That's a real problem here," Cochrane explained as the boy left. "These patients go anesthetic. They lose all sense of touch and pain, so we have to watch them carefully. They hurt themselves without knowing it." *How could anyone not notice a cut like that?* Paul thought to himself. From medical school, he knew that up to twenty-one thousand sensors of heat, pressure, and pain crowd together in a square inch of the fingertip. How could he feel no pain from such an injury? Yet the boy had indeed shown no sign of discomfort.

Chingleput Leprosarium

Meanwhile Paul Brand was settling into the daily routine of a missionary surgeon until Dr. Robert Cochrane, the indomitable Scotsman who had summoned him to India in the first place, upended that routine by inviting him to visit his leprosarium. Brand knew little about the disease in which Bob Cochrane had achieved world renown.

At the hospital in Vellore, Brand had often seen forlorn beggars with the deformities characteristic of leprosy. "Why don't you come to my clinic?" he asked these beggars. "At least we could examine you and dress your sores." "No, *daktar*, we could never come," they responded. "No hospital would let us in. We are lepers." He checked with the hospital, and found that to be true. Vellore, like every other general hospital in India, had a strict policy against admitting leprosy patients for fear lepers would frighten away other patients. He put the matter out of mind—until Cochrane insisted he visit the leprosy sanatorium in Chingleput.

Besides overseeing daily operations at the thousand-patient leprosy sanatorium in Chingleput, Cochrane also served as temporary director of the Vellore medical college and headed up government leprosy programs for the entire state. Rising at five each morning, he worked nonstop even on the hottest summer days until ten in the evening, when he retired for an hour or two of Bible study.

Cochrane's war against leprosy amounted to a religious crusade. "I'm not interested in Christianity. I'm interested in Christ, which is an entirely different matter," he would say. Citing the example of Jesus, who had broken cultural taboos by reaching out to victims of leprosy, Cochrane led a campaign against the prevailing social stigma. He sent shock waves through the medical community by hiring leprosy patients ("burnt-out" cases he considered noninfectious) to work in his home as his personal cook and his gardener.

Most significantly, Cochrane pioneered the use of dapsone for the treatment of leprosy. Dapsone is the first and chemically the simplest of the sulfones developed in Germany, first used as an antibiotic in 1937. It prevents the multiplication of *M. leprae.*

The sanatorium run by the Church of Scotland had a sterling reputation. Leprosy patients tended to live apart from society, forming their own communities beside a garbage dump or some such remote place. Even leprosy institutions housed their patients in squalid compounds away from population centers. In contrast, Chingleput was a lovely, sprawling campus of neat yellow buildings with red tile roofs. Years before, missionaries had planted long rows of mango and tamarind trees and, as a result, Chingleput now stood out as an oasis in the rocky, red-clay terrain south of Madras.

On a mild, sunny day in 1947, Paul Brand finally visited Bob Cochrane at Chingleput. As the two strolled down a shady pathway, Cochrane filled the ear of the young surgeon with facts about leprosy. "It's hardly contagious at all," he said. "Only one in twenty adults is even susceptible—the rest couldn't contract it if they tried. Leprosy used to be terrible, but now, thanks to sulfone drugs, we can arrest the disease at an early stage. If we could just get society to catch up with advances on the medical front, we could shut this place down. Our patients could return to their communities and resume their lives."

In between these mini-lectures, Cochrane proudly showed off the cottage industries he had established: weaving, bookbinding and cobbler shops, vegetable gardens, and carpentry sheds. He seemed oblivious to the gargoylish appearance of the advanced leprosy patients, but Brand had to fight the temptation to avert his eyes from the more disfigured faces. Some had the so-called "leonine" characteristics of

leprosy: flattened noses, no eyebrows, and greatly thickened forehead and cheekbone areas. They had such little control over facial muscles that it was hard to distinguish a smile from a grimace. Brand noticed a red-stained, milky film on many eyes, and Cochrane informed him that leprosy often blinds its victims. *I wonder if Margaret could help with their eye problems*, Brand thought to himself.

Soon, however, the leprosy patients' hands had captured his full attention, for Brand had trained as a hand surgeon. Never had he seen so many stumps and claw-hands. Shortened fingers jutted out at unnatural angles, their joints frozen into position. Other fingers bent downward against the palm in a fixed claw position, with the fingernails actually indenting the flesh of the palm. Some hands lacked thumbs and fingers altogether.

"Bob, tell me about how leprosy affects bones," Brand said. "Look at the hands of that woman. She has no fingers left, just a stump. What happened to her fingers? Did they fall off?"

"Sorry, Paul, I don't know," he replied.

"Don't know! But Bob, these patients will need their hands for any kind of livelihood. Something's destroying the tissue. You can't just let those hands waste away."

Cochrane's eyebrows arched upward. "And who is the orthopedist around here, Paul!" he demanded. "I'm a dermatologist, and I've studied this disease for twenty-five years. I know most of what there is to know about how leprosy affects skin. But you go back to that medical library in Vellore and look up the research on leprosy and bones. I can tell you what you'll find—nothing! No orthopedist has ever paid attention to this disease, even though it's crippled twice as many people as polio or any other single disease."

Could it be true that not one of the thousands of orthopedic surgeons had taken interest in a disease that produced such terrible deformities? Cochrane responded as if he had read Brand's mind. "You're thinking of leprosy like other diseases," he said. "But doctors, like most people, put it in a separate category altogether. They view leprosy as a curse of the gods. It still has the aura of supernatural judgment about it. You'll find priests, missionaries and a few crackpots working in leprosy settlements, but rarely a good physician and never a specialist in orthopedics."

As they continued the tour, one man motioned for them to stop, then asked if they would look at a sore on his foot. He squatted on the ground and tried to unbuckle his sandal, but couldn't manage it with his hand pulled into a claw position. Every time he tried to slide the sandal strap between his thumb and palm in order to tug it free of the buckle, the strap slipped away. "Paralysis from nerve damage," Cochrane remarked. "That's what this disease does. Paralysis, plus complete anesthesia. This fellow can't feel his sandal strap any more than the boy at the loom could feel his cut finger."

Brand asked the sandal-wearer if he could examine his hands. The fingers were full-length and intact, but virtually useless. The thumb and four fingers curved in and pressed against each other in the position known as "leprosy claw-hand." As he examined the man's hand, to his surprise the fingers felt soft and supple, very unlike fingers made stiff through arthritis or other crippling diseases. Brand pried the fingers open and slipped his own hand between the bent thumb and fingers. "Squeeze," he said. "As hard as you can."

Anticipating a weak twitch from nearly paralyzed muscles, Brand was startled to feel a jolt of pain shoot through his own hand. This man had the grip of a body-builder! "Stop!" he cried, and looked up to see a puzzled expression on the man's face. *What a strange visitor*, he must have thought. *He asks me to squeeze hard, then yells when I do.*

Paul Brand felt more than pain in that moment. He felt a sudden awakening, a tiny prod signaling the beginning of a long, boundless search. He had the intuitive sense of stumbling on a path that would send his life in a new direction.

He had just spent a very depressing morning, seeing hundreds of hands that cried out for treatment. As a hand surgeon, he had shaken his head in sadness at the waste, for until this moment he had thought them permanently ruined. Now, in one man's grip he had firsthand proof that a useless hand concealed live, powerful muscles. Paralysis? His own hand still ached from his grip.

The man's puzzled look only added to the mystery. Until the doctor cried out, he had no idea he had hurt him. He had lost sensory contact with his own hand.

Accepting Cochrane's challenge, when Brand returned to Vellore he checked the literature on orthopedic aspects of leprosy. He learned that ten to fifteen million people worldwide were estimated to suffer from the disease. Since a third of them sustained significant damage to the hands and feet, leprosy quite possibly represented the single greatest source of orthopedic crippling. One source suggested that leprosy caused more hand paralysis than all other diseases combined. Yet he could find only one article describing any surgical procedures other than amputation, an article that bore the byline "Robert Cochrane."

⁓

By now Paul Brand's scientific instincts were fully aroused. Even severely afflicted leprosy patients retained some good nerves and muscles—as the man with the claw hand had demonstrated so powerfully—a fact which opened up the tantalizing possibility of surgical correction. A claw-hand patient could still bend his fingers inward; if he could figure out how to free them to straighten in an outward direction, the patient would regain a functioning hand.

Before proceeding, though, he had to learn much more. He read everything available about leprosy, soon discovering why Cochrane had become such a crusader. No disease in history has been so marked by stigma, much of it the result of ignorance and false stereotypes. Yet, as Cochrane had affirmed, such fear was largely unfounded.

A Calling Confirmed

The effect on a person's appearance was leprosy's main curse. Sores appeared on the face, hands, and feet; if left untreated, gangrene often set in. Fingers and toes mysteriously shortened in length. Beggars that Brand observed in the streets of India usually had raw, suppurating sores and deformed hands and feet. The more aggressive beggars would sometimes threaten to touch a passerby unless he or she gave alms.

He was not sure what contribution he could offer leprosy patients, but the more time he spent among them, the more confirmed Brand felt in his calling. While visiting Chingleput, he listened to wrenching stories of rejection and despair. Kicked out of homes and villages, the patients came to Chingleput because they literally had nowhere else to go. They had become social outcasts simply because of their misfortune in contracting a feared and misunderstood disease. For the first time, Brand grasped the human tragedy of leprosy. He had also caught a whiff of hope that progress could be made in reversing that tragedy.

He set up a weekly visit to Chingleput, organizing an assembly-line team of technicians that examined one by one the thousand patients at Chingleput. Testing with a feather and a straight pin, the team mapped sensitivity to touch and pain in the various regions of the hand. Then they measured the range of movement of thumb, fingers and wrists, and repeated the procedure for toes and feet. They recorded the precise length of fingers and toes, noting which digits had shortened and which muscles seemed to be paralyzed. The most interesting cases, they X-rayed.

After completing the research, Brand could hardly wait to attempt reconstructive surgery on claw-hands. There was a chance, just a chance, that by transferring the strength of the

Debilitating But Not Fatal

However it spreads, leprosy rarely affects more than one percent of the population of a given region. There are a few exceptions to that rule, and the area around Vellore, India, happened to be one of them; in the 1940s more than three percent of the surrounding population showed signs of leprosy.

Most infected patients have a good chance of fighting off the disease on their own. These "tuberculoid" cases may suffer patches of dead skin, the loss of sensation, and a little nerve damage, but no extensive disfigurement. Many of the symptoms result from the body's own furious auto-immune response to the foreign bacilli.

One in every five patients, however, lacks any natural immunities. These unprotected patients, classified "lepromatous," are usually the ones who end up in facilities like Chingleput. Their bodies seem to put out a welcome mat for the foreign invaders and trillions of bacilli lay siege in a massive infiltration that, were it by any other strain of bacteria, would mean certain death. But leprosy rarely proves fatal. It wrecks the body in slow, debilitating ways. Indian patients sometimes use a Tamil word for leprosy which literally means "creeping death."

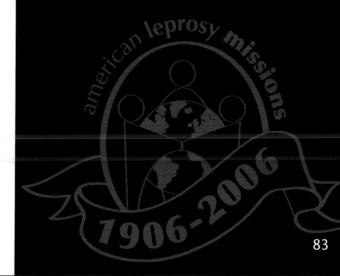

83

Learning from the Dead

Before trying some corrective hand surgery on patients with motor paralysis, Paul needed to know whether some muscles would remain "good," unaffected by the disease. Of course, he could not ethically operate on a living patient for the sole purpose of analyzing nerves. Autopsies were the only solution.

Alas, in India autopsies were more problem than solution. Moslem mullahs forbade bodily mutilation after death, even for the purpose of donating organs to science. The Hindu faith required that the entire body be burned to ashes in a purifying fire, and so very strict Hindus resisted amputation for any reason.

To meet its needs for organ transplants and laboratory work, the Vellore hospital sometimes used the bodies of dead prisoners and derelicts who had no families. (Margaret Brand, who had broadcast her need for eyes to use in corneal grafts, vividly remembers a knock on the door late one evening. She opened it to find a rather spectral figure shrouded in a cloth. He thrust before her a handwritten note from the local judge which she read by the light of his hurricane lantern: "Judicial hanging at dawn. Be there to get the eyes.")

At last a body became available, and Paul arrived with a dissection assistant at 2:30 a.m. to conduct the autopsy. He had promised the Chingleput superintendent they would complete the task by dawn, only four hours away. They hung the lantern from the roof beam, switched on a pocket flashlight for closeup work, and donned rubber aprons and gloves. The body had lain in an unventilated hut all day under a broiling sun and, to put it delicately, was fast moving toward a state of over-ripeness. The setting—a silent moonlit night, the heat, the isolation, a corpse full of germs—was worthy of a horror movie. That autopsy, though, provided key evidence that the disease always left certain muscles unaffected. As a hand surgeon, Paul could now identify forearm muscles for use in reconstructive surgery—possibly to transfer over to replace the paralyzed muscles—with no fear that they might become paralyzed later.

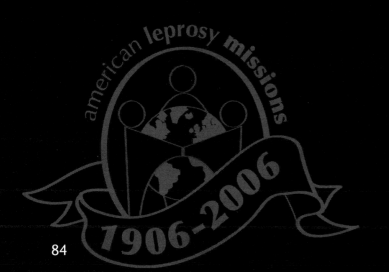

"good" muscles left untouched by leprosy, he could free clenched fingers and restore movement to damaged hands.

The Fear Barrier

When Brand sought the hospital's permission to perform such surgery, though, roadblocks went up. Even staff who were otherwise supportive could not countenance the Vellore hospital admitting leprosy patients. Nevertheless, after much lobbying the hospital did grant permission for Paul to open a Hand Research Unit—they dared not use the word leprosy—in a mud-walled storeroom attached to the outer wall of the hospital compound. Leprosy patients began streaming to the clinic.

As he began treating leprosy patients, Brand had to confront his own deep-seated prejudice and fear. Patients presented the most horrible, purulent sores for treatment, and often the pungent odor of pus and gangrene filled the storeroom. Even though he had heard Cochrane's assurances about the low contagion rate, he worried constantly about infection.

Margaret Brand led the way in overcoming the fear of close contact. One weekend when her husband was away, a cycle rickshaw pulled up to their house on the medical college campus. Out stepped a slim man in his early twenties. She noticed that his feet were heavily bandaged. White scars covered much of the surface of one eye, and he kept looking down to avoid the sun's glare. "Excuse me, Madam," the man said very respectfully, "could you tell me where I might find a Dr. Paul Brand?" She replied that her husband would not return until Tuesday, three days away. Obviously crestfallen, the man thanked her and turned to go. His rickshaw had already pulled off, so the man began walking back toward town in an awkward, hobbling gait.

She could not bear to turn away someone in need. Margaret Brand called to him. "You do have somewhere to go, don't you?" It took some coaxing, but in the next few minutes she managed to extract Sadan's story, an all-too-typical story of rejection and abuse. He had first noticed skin patches at the age of eight. Kicked out of school, he became a social outcast. His former friends crossed the street to avoid him. Restaurants and shops refused to serve him. After six wasted years, he finally found a mission school that would accept him, but after graduation no one would hire him. He managed to scrape together the fare for the train trip to Vellore. Once he arrived there, however, the driver of the public bus had refused to let him board. Sadan had then spent all his remaining cash to hire the rickshaw that brought him the four miles to the medical college. No, he had nowhere to go. Even if a hotel would let him in, he could not pay for the room.

In a flash Margaret Brand invited Sadan to sleep on the veranda of the Brands's home. She made a comfortable bed for him and he spent three nights there until Paul returned. Paul admitted that he did not react well when the children came rushing out to tell him about their new guest, the nice man with leprosy. His wife offered just this one-line explanation, "But, Paul, he had nowhere to go. . . ." Just that morning, she said, she had read the New Testament passage in which Jesus said, "For I was hungry and you gave me something to eat, I was thirsty and you gave me something to drink, I was a stranger and you invited me in, I needed clothes and you clothed me, I was sick and you looked after me." In that spirit, she had invited Sadan into their home. Besides teaching them about their own exaggerated fears, Sadan became one of the Brands's dearest friends.

A few months after opening the Hand Research Unit, Paul Brand was examining the hands of a bright young man, trying to explain to him in broken Tamil that they could halt the progress of the disease, and perhaps restore some movement to his hand, but they could do little about his facial deformities. He joked a bit, laying his hand on the patient's shoulder. "Your face is not so bad," Brand said with a wink, "and it shouldn't get any worse if you take the medication. After all, we men don't have to worry so much about faces. It's the women who fret over every bump and wrinkle." He expected a smile in response, but instead the man began to shake with muffled sobs.

"Have I said something wrong?" the doctor asked his assistant in English. "Did he misunderstand me?" She quizzed the patient in a spurt of Tamil and reported, "No, doctor. He says he is crying because you put your hand around his shoulder. Until he came here no one had touched him for many years."

Loosening the Claw

On his next trip to Chingleput, Brand assembled a group of leprosy patients who had been preselected for their advanced state of paralysis. He wanted volunteers whose hands he could not make worse. "In the hospital at Vellore, we are planning some experiments that *might possibly* help a paralyzed hand," he told them. "We need a few volunteers. The procedures have never been tried, and there is no guarantee whatsoever that they will work. You'll have to come to the hospital for a long stay involving several surgeries, and the rehabilitation process will be very strenuous. Again, we may find there's no improvement at all." He made the process sound as unappealing as possible in order to dampen expectations. Yet when he asked for volunteers, every patient stood up.

A Hindu teenager named Krishnamurthy was selected first. Leprosy had ravaged his hands and feet. He had large ulcers on the soles of both feet, exposing bone. His fingers, nearly their original length, curled in to form a stiff claw. He had a strong grasping motion but could not open his fingers enough to hold what it was he wanted to grasp. Every muscle in Krishnamurthy's hand was paralyzed, plus a few forearm muscles.

Cochrane insisted that Krishnamurthy was one of the brightest patients at Chingleput; he could, after all, read six languages. Leprosy, however, had broken his spirit. His dress was

ragged, his head hung low, and his eyes were blank and lightless. Mainly, he seemed interested in a free trip away from the sanatorium. Brand reiterated to him that his hand would probably need several different operations and he could make no guarantees. The boy shrugged and made a casual gesture, pulling the edge of one hand across his other wrist as if to say, "Cut it off if you wish. It's of no use to me."

The surgical team decided to employ a muscle in the forearm that normally helps bend the ring finger, transferring its tendon to a new site on the back of the thumb. The surgery lasted about three hours, much of it consumed by Brand's attempts to gauge how much tension to apply on the tendon. He used his best guess based on what he had learned from cadavers, then sutured the incisions, and wrapped the hand in a plaster splint.

For three weeks they waited. Without doubt Brand and the other medical staff were more nervous than Krishnamurthy himself on the day his bandages came off. He was the first leprosy patient in history to undergo such a procedure. Other physicians had groused that the team was wasting time trying to reverse progressive paralysis. Insensitive to pain, Krishnamurthy showed no signs of post-operative tenderness, and he let Brand move his fingers back and forth, up and down. The transplanted tendon seemed to be holding.

"You try it," the doctor said, in the final test. Krishnamurthy stared hard at the thumb, as if willing it to obey. It took his brain a few seconds to figure out a new pattern for thumb movement, but then it moved! Stiffly, minutely at first, but unmistakably. He grinned and the nurse beside him cheered aloud. Krishnamurthy wiggled his thumb again, basking in the spotlight.

Brand and the nurses could only imagine what was happening inside that hand. For years the teenager had worked to control his thumb. He had tried to pull it straight, using his other hand, but the thumb would always snap back into the clawed position before he could use it. It was a castoff, a vestigial appendage that neither moved nor felt sensation. Now, a part of his body long since given up for dead was coming back to life.

A few weeks later, Brand operated again, transplanting other tendons to help liberate Krishnamurthy's index and middle fingers. Progress came slowly, as laborious hours of physiotherapy had to follow each surgery. Until Krishnamurthy mastered independent finger movements his claw hand worked crudely, like a grasping hook worn by an amputee. He learned to hold a rubber ball, which he spent many hours squeezing, then a spoon, and even a pencil. After much practice, he could open and close his fingers at will, nearly forming a fist. One day he proudly demonstrated a new skill: he scooped up rice and curry from his food plate, formed it in a ball with the help of his opposing thumb, and dropped it in his mouth without spilling a single grain.

With each stride new aspects of Krishnamurthy's personality emerged. He laughed again, played practical jokes on the nursing staff, and scoured the hospital library for books he had not read. The light returned to his eyes. He became a Christian and adopted the Christian name "John." Before long he learned to type, and offered to translate some health materials into the local dialects. Passing by his room one morning to see him happily pecking away at a typewriter keyboard, Brand thought back to the bedraggled beggar boy who had once cowered like a wounded animal, his hands hanging useless at his side.

After the initial success, the hospital released two more isolation rooms for the use of indigent leprosy patients, and soon patients were filing in and out of the ward. A fine young surgeon named Ernest Fritschi joined Brand, and together the two of them explored any technique that held out some promise for restoring damaged hands.

By borrowing a strong muscle tendon from the forearm high above the normal region of paralysis, a muscle that had previously served to move the wrist, they found an improved way to correct the claw hand. Through a small incision near the wrist they pulled the tendon out, affixed a free graft from the leg, and tunneled the lengthened tendon all the way through the wrist and into the palm of the hand. Making another incision, they pulled the tendon out again, split it into four separate branches, and tunneled each branch to a different finger. The patient could then bend all four fingers simultaneously and straighten them where they had been clawed, utilizing the strength transferred from the powerful forearm muscle.

Meanwhile, Fritschi turned his attention to the foot. In a survey at Chingleput he found that large numbers of patients suffered from "foot drop" due to paralysis in the muscles responsible for lifting the feet and toes. Each time one of these patients lifted a leg off the ground, the foot dropped and the heel would not go down. In time the Achilles tendon shortened, so that each step put enormous pressure on the downward-pointing toes. With the body's full weight coming down on the toes rather than on the heel designed to bear that weight, the skin broke down and sores developed. Adapting what they had learned about tendon transfers in the hand, the surgeons were able to correct this problem in the foot as well, and soon Chingleput began to see a marked decrease in foot ulcers.

Those were heady days at the humble Hand Research Unit. They suffered failures, of course, such as a patient who threw himself in a well after learning that the team could do nothing to save two of his fingers. But since they drew from a patient base of gross deformities and defects, most procedures brought about a significant improvement. The patients themselves seemed honored that a medical team would lavish such care on them. Even if their hands and feet improved only slightly, almost always they left Vellore with a new enthusiasm and hope.

The Silent Destroyer

Father Damien, the Belgian priest in Hawaii, knew for certain he had leprosy when, shaving one morning, he spilled a mug of scalding water over his foot and felt no pain. That was in 1885. Leprosy workers had long recognized that the disease silenced pain signals, leaving the patient vulnerable to injury. Yet patients and health workers alike believed that leprosy caused even worse damage directly. Leprous flesh rotted away and died.

The more Paul Brand worked with leprosy patients, though, the more he questioned that common view of "bad flesh." He learned early on that the scenes depicted in popular novels and movies (*Papillon, Ben Hur*) were misleading; the limbs and appendages of leprosy patients do not simply drop off. Patients lost their fingers and toes over a long period of time, as his studies confirmed. Hand X-rays revealed bones that had mysteriously shortened, apparently from sepsis, with the skin and other soft tissues shrinking back to the length of bone. Something was causing the body to consume its own finger from the inside.

When he began the tendon transfer surgeries in the Hand Research Unit, Brand was still haunted by other physicians' predictions that these efforts would ultimately fail. Although patients might realize some short-term benefits from the surgery, skeptics predicted that the fingers so painstakingly corrected would eventually rot away as a result of leprosy's "bad flesh." If so, Brand and his colleagues were squandering valuable staff time and cruelly raising the hopes of patients.

Sadan, the gentle young man who had slept on the Brands's veranda, heightened these concerns. The surgeons had good success with his hands, and after a few months of surgery and recuperation Sadan landed a job as a clerk/typist. But nothing they tried seemed to help his feet. He had come to Vellore as a last resort after several doctors had advised amputation of both legs below the knee. His feet had shortened almost by half, and an angry red ulcer persisted on the ball of each rounded, toeless foot. The medical staff experimented with ointments, magnesium sulfate, penicillin cream, and any other treatment that might help clear up the ulcers, which in response only seemed to get worse. Sadan asked the team to stop wasting time on his feet. "Go ahead and amputate them as the other doctors recommended," he said.

One day Brand changed Sadan's dressings for at least the tenth time. Knowing that Sadan clung to him as a final hope, it broke his heart to tell him that the other doctors were probably right. The feet might have to come off because the clinic could not stop the spread of infection. Sadan received the news with sad resignation.

Instead of returning to the examining room, Brand stood and watched Sadan walk down the steps, cross a sidewalk, and head down the road. For the first time he noticed something: Sadan had no limp! Sadan had just spent half an hour in the clinic getting treatment for a grossly abscessed wound on the ball of his foot, and now he was putting his full weight on the exact same spot. No wonder the wound never healed! Gentian violet, penicillin, and every drug in the dispensary stood no chance of helping Sadan as long as he, quite unintentionally and due to his lack of pain, kept the tissue in a continual state of trauma. At last Brand had found the culprit responsible for the non-healing wound: the patient himself.

Dr. Ernest Fritschi came up with the best solution. "We use plaster casts on our hand patients and their surgical wounds heal properly," he said. "Why don't we apply the same treatment to foot ulcers?" This simple idea proved more valuable than all the other treatments put together. Three or four months' rest inside hard plaster sufficed to heal the stubbornest ulcers. Like a medieval knight's armor, the full-limb plaster gave a hard shell of protection for tender tissue. Pain-sensitive patients needed no such protection, for the vanguard of pain would never let them rest their body weight on an ulcerous foot as Sadan had done.

The amputation rate among leprosy patients at Vellore began to drop dramatically. Other doctors at the hospital, skeptical of the work with leprosy patients, expressed astonishment at these results. Where was the "bad flesh" of leprosy?

Brand berated himself for not identifying the problem sooner. Medical training had taught him to attune to patients' complaints about pain, but nothing had prepared him for the unique plight of people who do not feel pain. He had no idea how vulnerable the body becomes when it lacks a warning system. Working with patients such as Sadan triggered a revolution in his thinking about pain. He had long recognized its value in informing the brain of injury after the fact, but had no real appreciation for the many loyal ways in which pain protects *in advance*. Healing ulcers proved to be a simple matter compared to preventing them in the first place among those who lacked this advance warning system.

The surgical team was still working on the problem of foot ulcers when a potentially devastating problem surfaced among their first hand surgery patients. Some returned to the clinic with the dismaying news that their newly mobile fingers were still shortening. Chagrined, for they knew how much time and effort the Hand Research Unit had devoted to their care, they confessed that their fingers were developing sores and ulcers at a faster rate now than before the surgery.

Brand's heart sank as he examined their newly injured hands. "Don't waste your energy on leprosy, Paul," colleagues had warned him. Perhaps they were right. What good was a surgically-reconstructed hand if the patient ended up destroying it anyway? The clinic would dress the wounds and wrap them in plaster of paris. Months later the same patients returned with new signs of tissue damage.

The pattern perplexed the Vellore staff for months and threatened to derail the entire leprosy

Every Patient Has a Story

In lobbying for experimental treatment, Paul Brand told other hospital staff about some of the leprosy patients he had met. In a nation with a five-thousand-year tradition of caste, leprosy victims occupied the lowest rung of the social ladder. Their own families usually evicted them, with good reason: otherwise, the village would run the entire family out of town.

He examined one young boy with nodules all over his body who had been locked in an upstairs room for seven years. Before coming to the Chingleput sanatorium, another teenager had kept his left hand in his pocket to hide the telltale skin patches: below the tan line his hand was soft and pale like a baby's, and very weak from disuse.

Leprosy strikes twice as many males as females—no one knows why—but in India, Paul heard the most poignant stories from young girls who contracted the disease. Unable to find husbands or jobs, many of them ended up begging on the streets, assigned to a patch of pavement by a gang chieftain who exploited their earnings. Some served time in a brothel until the disease became noticeable to customers.

One objection to admitting leprosy patients probably lay at the root of the staff resistance. "If word got out that we were treating lepers here," an administrator said bluntly, "other patients would flee the hospital in fear. We can't risk that. Why not go and treat leprosy in leprosy centers where it belongs?"

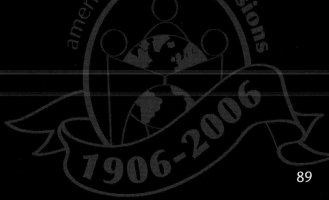

program. Before proceeding any further, they needed to find the cause of hand injuries, just as they had done with foot injuries. Brand decided to spend more time with rehabilitated surgical patients in order to observe their normal routine. Many of the teenage boys were now living in a makeshift village of mud huts and thatch roofs near Vellore. He asked these boys, about twenty-five in number, to try and help his team unravel the mystery of spontaneous wounds.

First the team made a baseline survey, tracing outlines of the boys' hands on a piece of paper and noting every scar or sign of finger damage. For weeks, even months, Brand visited them nearly every day, examining and measuring their hands, watching them work and play, studying every minor abnormality. It did not take long to discover why boys who had managed to stay free of injuries before surgery sometimes got into more trouble afterward. With new mobility and strength, they subjected their hands to more risk.

Some culprits he spotted right away. One young man was working as a carpenter. He had left the clinic in high spirits several months before, proud that his once-paralyzed fingers could again curl around the handle of a hammer, thrilled to resume an occupation he had thought lost to him forever. Brand was equally excited that the boy had found a source of income. But neither doctor nor patient had foreseen the hazards of carpentry without pain.

When a large blister appeared on the boy's hand, Brand easily matched it to a splinter on the hammer handle: he had pounded away all day with a wood splinter sticking in the flesh of his palm. The doctor fashioned a thicker, padded handle for his hammer, solving the splinter problem. Then he noticed the boy's fingertips beginning to show signs of abuse, so he taught him to hold nails with a pair of pliers.

Each occupation had distinct dangers. One young farmer used a hoe all day, not noticing a nail that stuck out from its handle into his palm. Another boy damaged his hand on a spade with a cracked handle that had been wrapped in baling wire. A barber lost his ring finger and nearly his middle finger due to the repetitive pressure of working a pair of scissors. A few simple design changes made these tools safer as well.

One of the most careful patients, a boy named Namo, experienced his first major setback when he volunteered to hold a floodlight for an American visitor who dropped by to shoot film footage of the leprosy work. Insensitive to heat, Namo didn't notice when the floodlight handle began to get hot due to cracks in the insulation. As soon as he set the light down, though, he saw shiny pink blisters forming on his hands. He dashed out of the room and Brand followed him. Without thinking he asked, "Namo, does it hurt?"

Namo gave a poignant reply. "You know it doesn't hurt me!" he cried. "I'm suffering in my mind because I can't suffer in my body."

All this time, as Paul Brand was tracking injuries, a suspicion grew in his mind. One day

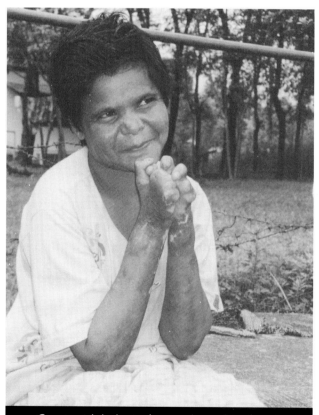

Constant injuries to leprosy-insensitive hands have maimed Harini's fingers and made her a victim of stigma and rejection by others.

he shared his idea with the patients. "We've seen that the people who talk about the 'bad flesh' of leprosy are wrong. Your flesh is as good as mine. The problem is that you don't feel pain and so it's easy for you to injure yourselves. You've already been very helpful in identifying the cause of many hand injuries. I have a theory I'll need your help to test. What if we assume that *all* wounds occur because of accidents—not because of leprosy itself?"

He asked the patients to join the team in a detective hunt: together they would track down the cause of every single injury. They would meet as a group weekly, and each boy would have to accept responsibility for his injuries. Never could anyone say about a wound, "It just came by itself," or, "That's what leprosy does." If he detected a new blister on the back of a knuckle or a spot of inflammation on the thumb, he wanted some explanation, no matter how far-fetched it sounded.

Some of the boys hid their wounds at first. Years of rejection had conditioned them to conceal injuries, and they found it shameful to acknowledge their wounds so openly. In contrast, those who became known as the "naughty boys" seemed to take morbid delight in their painlessness. One boy pushed a thorn through the palm of the hand until it poked through the other side like a sewing needle. Sometimes Brand felt like a schoolmaster, with the odd sense that he was introducing the boys to their own limbs, begging their minds to welcome the insensitive parts of their bodies.

As weeks went by, the message finally sank in and the group joined together in the detective hunt. Whenever a wound appeared, the team examined it in search of a cause, then applied a splint to keep the finger or hand out of action until it had healed. They uncovered both everyday and exotic causes of spontaneous wounds, feeling especially proud when they managed to solve a difficult case. Once the staff and patients had ferreted out the origin of an injury, they could usually prevent it from reoccurring.

Over time, Paul Brand's team, working closely with the patients, learned to account for 90 percent of spontaneous wounds. By far the most mystifying injuries involved the sudden disappearance of almost a whole segment of a finger or toe. Every once in a while a leprosy patient would show up at the daily meetings and sheepishly display a raw, bleeding patch, with the flesh around an inch-length section of a finger or big toe missing and bare bone exposed. This oddity defied everything they had learned about the disease and, unless the mystery was solved, it put the entire theory of painlessness in jeopardy. To other hospital personnel, it would confirm the worst myths about leprous fingers and toes "falling off" due to bad flesh.

Almost always, the afflicted person noticed the missing digit in the morning. Something ominous was taking place during the night. In the end, a patient solved the mystery by sitting up all night in an observation post. He watched a scene straight out of a horror movie. In the middle of the night a rat climbed onto the bed of a fellow patient, sniffed around tentatively, nuzzled a finger and, meeting no resistance, began to gnaw on it. The lookout yelled, waking the whole room and scaring away the rat. At last they had the answer: the boys' fingers and toes had not dropped off—they were being eaten!

This most repugnant cause of spontaneous wounds had an easy remedy. First, the staff set traps for the rodents and built barriers around the beds of patients. When trouble continued, they settled on a more effective solution: they went into the cat breeding business, using the blood line of a proven Siamese male who was an excellent ratter. From then on, no leprosy patient could leave the rehabilitation center without a feline companion. The problem of missing pieces of fingers vanished almost overnight.

Retraining the Mind

Early on, Paul Brand performed a tendon transfer on a patient who, like John Krishnamurthy, had a paralyzed thumb and claw-hand paralysis. He performed the now-perfected operation, moving a tendon from the ring finger over to his thumb. Evidently, he had not explained the results carefully enough to him. When nurses unwrapped the bandages several weeks after surgery Paul said to him, "Now you can bring your thumb forward." The patient struggled, with a look of some consternation on his face, for the surgeon had promised him a movable thumb and nothing was happening. He was unable to get any movement at all out of that thumb.

"Well, try your ring finger," Paul said. The patient's thumb leaped forward and he jumped backward! The two laughed together, and the surgeon explained that he would have to retrain his brain to think *thumb* instead of *ring finger*. They had confused the brain by, in effect, rewiring the motor nerves. For days afterward he sat on a mat, studying his thumb, wiggling it, remapping the neural pathways in his brain. Ultimately the team had to stop performing radical tendon transfers for leprosy patients over the age of forty. If they tried to convert muscles to perform a completely new task, the older patients' brains could not make the reprogramming adjustments.

Paul Brand began leprosy work with a singular desire to repair damaged hands. Along the way he met with an even greater challenge: quite simply, to keep leprosy patients from destroying themselves. New dangers sprang up, Hydra-like, to replace those eliminated. Lists of rules for the patients were posted: Never walk barefoot. Inspect your hands and feet every day. Don't smoke (nurses frequently had to treat "the kissing wound," named for the adjacent burn marks a cigarette leaves if held too long between insensitive fingers). Wrap hot objects with a cloth. When in doubt, wear gloves. Use coconut oil to soften skin and prevent cracks. Don't eat in bed (so as not to attract rats and ants). On a bus or truck, don't sit near the hot engine or rest your feet on a metal floor. Always use a mug modified with a wooden handle.

In time the tide of battle turned, and the incidence of spontaneous wounds plummeted. Indeed, the most conscientious patients now kept their hands and feet free of any serious damage. Even the most reluctant patients, those who had joined the group solely as a favor to the staff, caught the vision. More than promoting a cold, scientific theory, the little group at Vellore was fighting a crusade to help overturn ancient prejudice against leprosy. Sulfone drugs could arrest the disease; perhaps proper care could prevent the deformities that made it so feared.

For most people, preventing avoidable injuries takes no conscious thought. The pain reflex will jerk a hand away from a hot object, order a limp if shoes fit too tight, and startle a sleeper awake if a rat even nuzzles a hand. Deprived of that reflex, leprosy patients must anticipate consciously what might harm them. Yet the conscious mind can do wonders. Constant harping on the dangers got results: at the end of one year, the Vellore team determined that not one finger had shortened among the boys in the experiment.

Brand had asked his patients to assume, just for the sake of the "detective hunt," that all damage to hands and feet was related to their insensitivity to pain. They had become so skilled

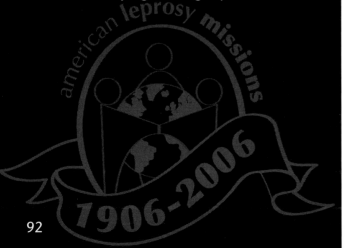

at tracking the causes of injury that he was now ready to go public with the radical theory that painlessness was the real enemy. Leprosy merely silenced pain, and further damage came about as a side effect of painlessness—which meant that all such damage was preventable.

He knew such a notion flew in the face of hundreds of years of tradition, and the medical community would likely greet a new theory with skepticism. But his patients had convinced him that painlessness, not leprosy, was the villain. The team at Vellore could now identify the underlying cause of virtually all injuries, and all were secondary effects. They had removed forever the most common excuse of patients: "The wound happened all by itself. It's just part of leprosy."

If he was right, the worldwide approach to leprosy treatment only addressed half the problem. Arresting the disease through sulfone drug treatments was not nearly enough; health workers also needed to alert leprosy patients to the hazards of a life without pain. He now understood why even a "burnt-out case" with no active bacilli continued to suffer disfigurement. Even after leprosy had been "cured," without proper training patients would continue to lose fingers, toes, and other tissue, because that loss resulted from painlessness.

Eyebrows and Noses

A young man named Kumar came to the center one day presenting a certificate that declared his leprosy inactive. The team at Vellore had worked on his hands, which now showed no sign of clawing or accidental injury, and his feet no sign of nerve paralysis. Paul Brand could spot only one visual reminder of the disease, naked patches where his eyebrows once grew, and these hardly seemed worth noting.

"Why have you come?" the doctor asked, after completing the examination. "As you know, we specialize in surgery of the hands and feet, and yours seem fine." Kumar pointed to his eyebrows, or rather the places on his face where eyebrows used to grow, and told his story.

Before contracting leprosy Kumar had tended a stall in the marketplace of his village. Village people are often shrewder than doctors at detecting the early signs of leprosy, and when Kumar's skin began to show an unnatural sheen, customers spread the news and trade dropped off. Before long, nobody bought his goods and few would even stop to talk. Kumar, too proud to become a beggar, closed down his stall and headed for a nearby leprosarium.

When he returned to the village several years later, negative health certificate in hand, he assumed he could resume his trade. All signs of the disease had vanished except the naked eyebrows. For superstitious village folk, though, this feature alone was enough to ostracize him. A certificate did not matter. He had to look free of the disease. He had to grow eyebrows.

"No one will buy from a man without eyebrows," Kumar reported sadly. "Please, Doctor, can you make me some eyebrows? I can't stand having customers peer at me and look for hairs to see if I'm really clean."

Brand listened to Kumar with mixed emotions. Although moved by Kumar's story, he certainly had no desire to get into cosmetic surgery. In view of the waiting list of candidates for corrective surgery, many of them with paralyzed hands that could be set free, a request for new eyebrows seemed almost trivial. And yet he remembered the lesson learned from other patients. Unless he could find a way to restore patients to a useful life in their villages, he would create a permanent class of dependents. If facial appearance created a barrier to acceptance, he had to find a way to knock it down.

Kumar stayed at Vellore a few days while Brand researched plastic surgery techniques that might help him. One procedure involved transferring eyebrow-shaped pieces of scalp to a new location. A successful transplant would guarantee Kumar eyebrows as bushy as the thick black hair on his head. Paul explained the process, and the patient enthusiastically consented.

The trick was to find a piece of scalp connected to blood vessels long enough to reach down to the eyebrow site. Before the surgery he clipped Kumar's hair very short and made him go for a run. Fifteen minutes later, when he climbed the stairs to the doctor's office, his heart was pounding and Paul could see arteries throbbing under his scalp. Using a marker, Paul traced the outline of his temporal artery, selected some long branches, and drew in two bold, wide eyebrow shapes, one on each side of his shaved head.

The next day Kumar lay on the wooden operating table as Brand cut out the eyebrow shapes he had marked and lifted them free of the skull. Still attached to an artery and vein, they hung down like two mice dangling by their tails. Next he removed the skin where Kumar's old eyebrows had been and made tunnels under the skin from each eyebrow up toward the opening in the scalp. Using long forceps he reached through the tunnel, grasped the dangling sections of scalp, and carefully pulled them to their new sites crowning Kumar's eyes. Transplanted, the scalp sections looked so large that he was tempted to trim them a bit, but feared cutting into the curving arteries that would keep the new eyebrows alive.

Brand need not have worried about their size. From the instant his dressings were removed, Kumar was delighted with his new eyebrows. As the hair began to grow, and kept on growing, his delight increased. Before he left Vellore, bushy eyebrows hung down over his eyes. Eventually, of course, Kumar did trim his eyebrows. But in his home village their very luxuriance created a sensation. Former customers lined up to have a look at Kumar's eyebrows, and this time when he showed them his certificate of cure from leprosy, they believed him.

The experience with Kumar's eyebrows opened up a whole new arena for corrective surgery: the face. Noses posed the next challenge. Bald eyebrow patches were a minor problem compared to the "saddleback noses" that disfigured many patients.

Because leprosy bacilli prefer cool areas, the nose becomes a major battleground. The body's response to the invaders causes inflammation which, if it persists, may block the airways. In time the mucus lining ulcerates from secondary infections, and the nose may shrink away to almost nothing. The elevated ridge of cartilage disappears, leaving a collapsed patch of skin and two flared nostrils that open directly outward. It is rather disconcerting, to say the least, to look at a leprosy face and see into a person's nasal cavities.

Everyone in India recognized the collapsed nose as a sign of leprosy—some believed that noses "rotted off" like toes and fingers—and any person so afflicted faced a life of stigma and ostracism. A woman with such a nose stood no chance of marriage, even if she was certified negative and bore no other marks of the disease.

After getting mixed results forming new noses with skin transplants from the forehead, the team at Vellore learned a new technique from Sir Harold Gillies, a plastic surgeon visiting from England. Gillies had observed that leprosy imbeds in the mucous lining of the nose and damages the inside lining of the nose much more severely than it damages the skin. Cartilage gets destroyed due to the resulting inflammation, and without cartilage to support it the expanse of skin collapses like a tent without poles. "Why bother to transplant skin when you have perfectly good skin sitting there unused?" Gillies asked. "The mucous lining has been destroyed, but you can always replace that with grafts once you reshape the nose."

They prepped a patient for surgery. Looking at his shrunken nose, Brand found it hard to imagine that anything worthwhile could be salvaged from that shriveled patch of skin. Gillies picked up a scalpel and demonstrated. Peeling back the upper lip, he cut inside the mouth between teeth and gum and lip until he could lift the lip high enough to expose the nasal cavity. He freed the whole upper lip and then the nose from its attachment to facial bones. "Now watch," he said. He took a roll of gauze and stuffed it inch by inch into the cavity of the shrunken nose. As if by magic the skin spread apart, stretched, and plumped up to form a quite respectable nose. Gillies assured the Vellore staff that if properly supported the nose would retain its new shape.

Over the next few years the Vellore team experimented with various supporting structures. They used nose-shaped plastic splints, then acrylic, then bone grafts from the pelvic rim. For those patients who had insufficient blood supply in the nasal tissue to sustain a bone graft, they borrowed material from dentists. They learned to fashion a soft warm mold of wax to virtually any shape. The patient, awake, could choose his or her nose on the spot: "A touch longer and not quite so wide, please." From that wax model they formed a permanent support made out of the hard pink substance used for dentures. Dental wire attached to the teeth held the structure in place.

Like the transplanted eyebrows, artificial noses had an immediate effect on the patients' social acceptance. One very pretty young woman came to Vellore with no marks or nodules on her face, but a fully collapsed nose. Her family had tried earnestly to find a groom for her, to no avail. She chose exactly the nose she wanted, a fine, dainty nose which she assured the team was much better looking than the original. A few months later she sent a photo of herself dressed up in wedding finery. Her disease had been cured; now the stigma was healing as well.

Today, many leprosy patients in India and around the world walk around with noses that look perfectly normal from the outside but are supported by an artificial under-nose insert. The new noses serve patients well as long as they follow a rather bizarre maintenance procedure: they must take out the artificial support periodically for cleaning in order to remove foreign matter and guard against infection. The gap between upper lip and jaw does not re-close, and it is a simple matter for the patient to peel back the upper lip and slide out the bright pink support material. The outer nose collapses back into its flattened, wrinkled shape, only to expand again when the clean under-nose is inserted.

Preventing Blindness

All this time, as the Vellore team perfected ways to reconstruct hands and feet and improve their patients' facial appearance, one of leprosy's worst afflictions went neglected: blindness. Old-timers insisted that blindness, like paralysis and tissue destruction, was a tragic but unavoidable consequence of the disease. In fact, leprosy experts estimate that leprosy is still the fourth-leading cause of blindness in the world.

Blindness presents an unusual hardship for leprosy patients who have also lost the sense of touch and pain. It may take a blind patient with insensitive fingers an hour to dress, for he or she must bend over the clothing and touch it with still-sensitive lips and tongue, feeling out the location of sleeves and buttons and buttonholes. A person both blind and insensitive also cannot read Braille, or learn a friend's face by touching it with fingertips, and will have difficulty maneuvering through a room crowded with furniture. An everyday task like cooking becomes almost impossible for someone who can neither see nor feel the dangers.

Without doubt, blindness is the most feared complication of leprosy. One Vellore patient, who had already lost sight in one eye, said quite openly, "My feet have gone and my hands too, but that didn't matter much as long as I could see. Blindness is something else. If I go blind, life will mean nothing to me and I shall do all I can to end it."

Margaret Brand made the first systematic study of the onset of blindness in leprosy patients. In the early days, as her orthopedic-surgeon husband was devoting himself to the subject of leprosy, she knew little about the disease's effect on eyes. It was while working on one of the cataract "eye camps" that she first became aware of the eye problems of leprosy patients. She recalled:

> I had just finished the active surgery and was loading equipment in the van for our trip

home, when I noticed a group of people sitting on the ground about forty yards away. I asked one of the workers if they were patients who had come late and needed attention. "Oh, those are just lepers," he said, and continued working. I offered to examine them anyway, much to my assistant's—and the patients'—surprise.

I had seen all sorts of eye problems in India, but never in my life had I seen eyes like these. The surface of the eye, normally moist and transparent, was clouded over with thick layers of white scar tissue. It looked like washed leather. I shone a penlight into the eye and got no response whatever. Most of these people were totally, irremediably blind. Two of the younger ones were well on the way but not quite blind, and the fully blind ones clung to them. I persuaded these two to come to Vellore with me for hospitalization.

From that one encounter, Margaret Brand's life work began to take shape. She learned that about 40 percent of leprosy patients would sooner or later suffer eye involvement, many developing blindness. Yet almost no one in the field had studied this facet of the disease. She opened an eye clinic devoted solely to the problem of ocular leprosy. The examination room was painted black, its windows covered with drapes, so that Brand could examine eyes in a dark environment.

Many patients presented with bad corneal ulcers. She would ask what happened to the eye, and they had no clue. "It just came." But by watching them, she could see what happened. Normally, if you get irritation in an eye, you close the eye and give it a gentle rub. Leprosy patients don't even close their eyelid; they put their finger on the tender spot and give it a good hard rub, tearing the delicate "skin" of the cornea while infecting it with germs from fingers—a sure recipe for an ulcer. She had one patient with a huge callus over the

base of his palm, which he used to rub his itchy eye. He then wondered why he went blind.

Brand also found that leprosy bacilli liked to gather in the cornea, one of the coolest parts of the body, but that temporary measures could help slow the damage to the eye. The body's defensive reactions against the bacilli produced tiny protein deposits called "iris pearls." In some cases, cortisone drops helped control this defensive reaction. In others, the damage could be surgically repaired. Also, by tattooing small droplets of India ink into the white scar tissue on the cornea, she could reduce the bright glare that tormented some leprosy patients.

All these measures, however, paled beside the most important observation Brand made as she surveyed hundreds of leprosy patients: many were going blind from not blinking.

The blink reflex is one of the wonders of the human body. No pain sensors are more sensitive than those on the surface of the eye: a stray eyelash, a speck of dirt, a flash of light, a puff of smoke or even a loud noise will trigger an instantaneous muscular response. The eyelid slams shut, pulling a protective skin covering over the vulnerable eye and trapping any foreign particles in the eyelashes.

Even more impressive, the intermittent blink reflex operates at a maintenance level all day long, opening and closing the eyelid every fifteen seconds or so to assure that the eye stays lubricated. The splendid mixture of oil, mucus, and watery fluid that we know as tears provides the cornea with a constant supply of nourishment and cleansing. Without that lubrication, the surface of the cornea dries out and becomes much more susceptible to damage and ulceration.

Brand noticed that some leprosy patients never bothered to blink at all. They had a relentless, unsettling stare, and their tears gathered in a pool in the lower lids until they spilled over. In the dusty atmosphere of India, a trail of wasted tears ran down the faces of these leprosy patients, their corneal cells deprived of the windshield-washer benefit of a blinking eyelid.

Over time, opaque scar tissue would replace the clear membrane.

She found that leprosy interfered with the blink reflex in two ways. Due to nerve damage, some leprosy patients (about 20 percent) experienced total paralysis of the eyelid muscle, almost overnight losing the motor ability to blink. These patients slept with their eyes wide open, and in time the cornea dried out and began to deteriorate.

Brand learned, though, that many more patients suffered from the familiar nemesis of painlessness. Try to go without blinking and after a minute or so you will feel a mild irritation. Keep your eyes open, and that irritation will gradually turn into intense pain, forcing you to blink. Pain first whispers, then shouts. Insensitive leprosy patients, however, do not perceive these pain signals. Just as the bacilli damage nerves in fingertips and toes, they also damage the hair-trigger pain sensors that provoke blinking. Numbed, those exquisite pain sensors on the surface of the eye never initiate the blink reflex.

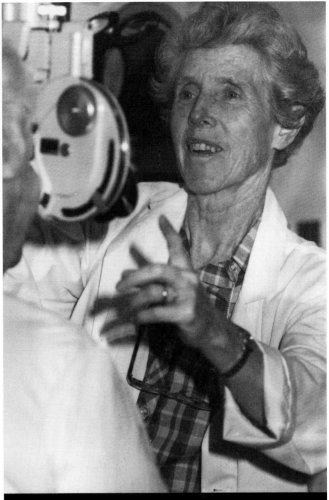

Dr. Margaret Brand examining a patient's eyes

Margaret Brand's research confirmed that most leprosy blindness was not an unavoidable consequence of infection but rather a byproduct caused by a breakdown in the nerves. She chose to work first with the insensitive patients who had not lost their motor nerves. For this large group, the solution seemed simple: she needed only to examine them regularly and train them to blink consciously rather than by reflex. If she educated the younger patients to the danger, surely they could learn to blink every minute or so. The alternative was blindness.

With great hope, Brand began an education campaign among these patients, drilling them to blink every time she held up a flashcard. They followed her lead enthusiastically for an hour or two, but later in the day as she walked among them she noticed the same wide-eyed, unblinking stare. She tried egg-timers, buzzers, and other timing devices. These too worked for a while, but patients either lost interest or became inured to the signal. She put goggles on the patients to protect their eyes against foreign objects, but still they were missing the essential benefits of blinking.

In desperation, the Vellore team researched surgical procedures that might help. Gillies had devised an elegant technique to aid people with Bell's palsy, who also have problems with the blinking muscle. His innovative procedure held out promise even for those with complete eyelid paralysis. It involved detaching one end of part of the temporalis muscle, which controls clenching of the jaw and chewing, and connecting it to a strand of fascia running through the eyelids. This adjustment made it easier for patients to blink consciously, for now the same muscle controlled both the motion of chewing and lid-closing.

Brand only had to teach her patients to clench their teeth periodically—or, better yet, chew gum—and the eye would get the lubrication it needed.

The procedure worked well, and is still used widely in India. If a patient chews gum vigorously every time he or she goes outdoors on a dusty day, the eye will get the protection it needs. The surgery produces some unusual side effects—a person blinks rapidly as she chews on a piece of meat—but a conscientious patient can keep blindness at bay simply by chewing.

Alas, never underestimate the contribution of pain. Solving the motor problems and thus restoring a patient's ability to blink did not solve the much more difficult sensory problems. Even her most eager patients, who held within their conscious power the ability to forestall blindness, would lapse. Unless they retained some residual pain sensation on the surface of the eye to alert them to a feeling of soreness or dryness, they would forget to blink or chew. They needed the compulsion of pain; for them to blink with perfect regularity, it had to hurt.

When a patient lacked all sensation of pain, surgeons had to revert to a much less satisfactory procedure. Using thread and needle, they stitched the upper and lower eyelids tightly together in the corners, leaving enough of an opening in the center to permit vision. Because so little of the eye was exposed, lubricating tears collected around the cornea and bathed it even though the patient never blinked. Patients hated the squinty effect on their appearance, as they hated anything that made them look unnatural, but at least it preserved their sight. Even today, this simple procedure, albeit a poor substitute for silenced pain cells, serves as a remarkable sight-saver for leprosy patients.

More than anything else, however, Brand found that leprosy treatment programs must include regular eye examinations by trained experts. Lacking the warning system of pain, leprosy patients had to rely on others to detect problems in early stages. The same principle Paul Brand had found in working with feet and hands, Margaret Brand found in working with eyes.

The Birth of Karigiri

The Brands's work with leprosy patients gradually overwhelmed other duties at the hospital. Often they lay awake at night discussing the patients, many of whom had become friends. What new surgical innovations might reduce the stigma they faced? How could they improve the quality of their lives? More and more, leprosy work became for both Brands a vocation, not mere avocation.

At a critical time, Paul Brand received a generous and quite unexpected offer from the Rockefeller Foundation. "Your work with leprosy shows good potential," their representative told him. "Why don't you travel around the world and get the best advice possible. See anyone you want—surgeons, pathologists, leprologists—and take whatever time you need. We'll foot the bill."

The Rockefeller-sponsored trip accomplished nearly everything he had hoped. Most important, it taught him how leprosy does its damage. He learned this from Dr. Derek Denny-Browne, a fellow Englishman and a brilliant neurologist who practiced at a charity hospital in Boston.

As Brand showed specimens from the Chingleput autopsy, Denny-Browne recognized a pattern he had seen in experiments performed on cats years before. At last he located a dusty box of microscope slides, pulled them out, and put them side by side with the Chingleput nerve specimens. Under the microscope, they matched perfectly. Brand now had two independent demonstrations of the same pattern, a pattern no other neurologist had been able to identify.

"Well, now, that tells you something," Denny-Browne said with obvious pride. "Your leprosy nerves are being damaged by ischemia. Something's causing them to swell, and the nerve sheath [a fat-protein sleeve resembling the insulation around a wire] restricts the swelling.

Karigiri

The Schieffelin Leprosy Research and Training Centre (SLRTC) at Karigiri in the state of Tamil Nadu, South India, began in 1955. It was the fulfillment of a dream shared by Bob Cochrane, Paul Brand, and Herbert Gass.

SLRTC, or "Karigiri" was named after William J. Schieffelin, the first chairman of the American Leprosy Missions board of governors. It was cofounded by ALM and The Leprosy Mission of Great Britain. It began as an offshoot of the Christian Medical College and Hospital at Vellore, about fifteen kilometers distant, but later became an independent partner in the research and delivery of health care for people affected by leprosy.

The land upon which Karigiri sits is legendary: what was once a semi-arid expanse of land at the foot of Elephant Hill, is now a flower-covered oasis, rich with trees, plants, and a huge variety of bird life. Much of the transformation is attributed to the planting, work, and vision of Dr. Ernest Fritschi and his father, who is buried there.

The institution has flowered, as well. Karigiri has a two-hundred-bed hospital admitting one thousand leprosy patients annually, and a registry of more than forty thousand outpatients. It conducts research, and is a training center with courses for everyone from village leprosy workers to shoe makers to surgeons. Trainees come from all over India and from all over the world. Among its most famous teacher/practitioners until their retirements were Drs. Paul and Margaret Brand, world renowned for their achievements in the surgery and care of leprosy-affected hands and eyes.

Karigiri researchers have contributed vitally to the body of knowledge about this disease. Studies in both laboratories and in the field (such as the control projects in Gudiyatham) have greatly enhanced what is known today about diagnosis, treatment, and disability.

Karigiri's rehabilitation projects have empowered many leprosy-disabled adults to become creatively and financially engaged in cottage-industry weaving projects. Today many of the weavers' children are attending secondary schools and colleges, and realizing dreams once considered impossible.

Christian nurture is an integral part of Karigiri. ALM has contributed towards the support of Karigiri chaplains and a speaker system that enables daily worship services to be broadcast throughout the wards. The beautiful stone chapel, simple and serene, is a sanctuary for all who seek the presence of Christ.

Farm, dairy, shoe shop, video unit, guest houses, patient canteen, computerized records, outpatient clinics, schools, workshops, craft sales, and elder care—Karigiri, with its staff of three hundred, has grown like the trees and flowers that startle the visitor with their beauty and fragrance.

It is not the buildings, facilities, flowers, or trees, though, that define Karigiri's spirit, but the commitment to serving God and seeking an end to the stigma that leprosy-affected people have endured for ages.

In the poignant words of Usha Jesudasan, writer and wife of the late Dr. Kumar Jesudasan, a longtime physician at Karigiri, "Today every leprosy patient can be cured physically with drugs, but for many the scars, the fears still remain . . . The miracle of healing is that caused by touch, by compassion, by putting oneself in the sufferer's place. Two thousand years of discoveries, high technology, research, plans, and conferences can never replace that essential ingredient that Jesus left us with . . . a large dose of love administered with a tender touch."

—Susan S. Renault

What happens is that pressure inside the sheath becomes so tight that it squeezes shut the blood supply and causes ischemia. Like any tissue, a nerve will die if it's cut off from blood supply long enough."

For the first time, Brand had a sensible explanation of leprosy's assault on the nerve. As the leprosy bacilli invade nerves, the body reacts with a classic response of inflammation, causing the nerve to swell. Bacilli multiply, the body sends in reinforcements, and before long the expanding nerve presses against its sheath. Eventually the swollen nerve squeezes shut its own blood supply and dies, no longer able to carry the electric signals for sensation and movement.

As he peered through the microscope lens in Denny-Browne's cluttered office, some of the final pieces of the leprosy puzzle clicked into place for Paul Brand. For centuries medicine had focused on the visible harm that leprosy did to toes, fingers and face—hence the "bad flesh" myth. His own work with patients, as well as the Chingleput autopsy, had convinced him that the real problem lay elsewhere, in the nerve pathways, but until that moment he had not understood how the nerves got damaged. Denny-Browne's explanation of ischemia solved the puzzle.

At last Brand was beginning to gain an overall picture of leprosy as primarily a disease of the nerves. Bacilli do proliferate in cool places such as the forehead and nose, provoking a defensive response, but those invaders do mostly cosmetic damage. The truly devastating symptoms come about when bacilli invade nerves close to the skin surface. Each major nerve is a conduit for motor and sensory fibers, and a failure in the nerve affects both. Motor axons no longer carry messages from the brain, and the hand or foot or eyelid muscle becomes paralyzed; sensory axons no longer carry messages of touch, temperature and pain, and the patient becomes vulnerable to injury. When an injury does occur an infection often sets in, and the body's reaction may cause the bone to be destroyed or absorbed, resulting in shortened fingers and toes.

Brand thought back to his first contact with the victims of leprosy, the beggars in the streets of Vellore. Their symptoms—blindness, marred faces, paralyzed hands, stumpy fingers and toes, open ulcers under the feet—apparently pointed to a disease of the skin and extremities. It had taken him a long time to be more precise in assigning blame. Now he had confirmation that most of the gross deformities and dreaded symptoms of leprosy had the same cruel source: damaged nerves.

He returned from the Rockefeller-sponsored trip armed with new surgical skills and loaded with ammunition for his theories on painlessness, but he also brought back the sobering knowledge that the Vellore team was on its own in India. None of the top neuropathologists had ever studied leprosy-damaged nerves, and of the noted surgeons he visited, only one had ever worked with its victims. By default, Vellore itself was the pioneering outpost in the campaign for leprosy rehabilitation.

The program still lacked an important element: a full-scale leprosy hospital and dedicated research center. The state government offered a 256-acre site in a rural area called Karigiri, fourteen miles from the medical college. Brand felt dismay the first time he inspected this gravelly, parched site for the first time. Hot winds swept across the sere landscape, and as he stepped from the jeep they hit him in the face like exhaust from a blast furnace. *No one on earth would choose to live in such a blighted place*, he thought to himself. But leprosy patients rarely have the luxury of personal choice: neighbors had blocked several lovely sites closer to town. He accepted the land gratefully and broke ground. Plans called for an eighty-bed hospital, a well-equipped research laboratory, and a training facility.

Karigiri soon named Dr. Ernest Fritschi to the post of chief surgeon, a wise move for reasons beyond his medical skills. Fritschi's father, a Swiss agricultural missionary, had taught his son basic principles of botany and ecology, and

Fritschi now adopted the wasteland at Karigiri as his most challenging "patient." He built dirt trenches, contour dams, and percolation dams in an effort to control erosion and raise the water table. He sought out drought-resistant plants to stabilize the thin soil. He planted as many as a thousand trees a year, nourishing seedlings in his own house, transplanting them carefully, and watering them with a bullock-drawn water tanker.

Ever so gradually, Karigiri was transformed. At first the grey and white buildings of the research center stood stark and tall against the shimmering horizon of the desert. Over time, a lush green forest grew up to shield those buildings, lowering the ground temperature and taming the whipsaw winds. Birds returned, as many as a hundred different species.

The research work at Karigiri kept pace with the physical improvements. Indeed, in the next few years surgeons and physiotherapists from more than thirty countries found their way to the tiny backwater town in the desert of South India. They could study medicine and epidemiology elsewhere, but no other place offered practical experience in the surgery and rehabilitation of leprosy patients.

For those who knew Karigiri in the early days, what transpired in the desert looked like a miracle of nature, an oasis of beauty and new hope sprouting in a landscape of death. That transformation mirrored what also took place in many of the patients. Many had come barren of all hope. Loving care did for the human spirit what it had done for the land.

On to Carville

In 1965, after nearly twenty years in India, the Brands made the difficult decision to move on. Skilled Indian personnel had assumed control of most branches of the leprosy work and, since Paul spent several months each year traveling internationally, his ties to Karigiri had begun to loosen. The Brand family now

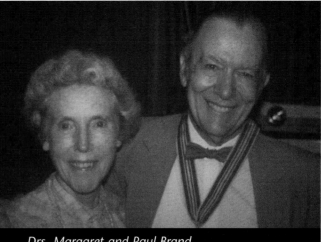

Drs. Margaret and Paul Brand

included six children, some nearing college age, and it seemed a good time for the family to relocate. They returned to England, expecting to make their permanent home there.

Those plans changed when a lecture tour took Paul Brand to the leprosy hospital in Carville, Louisiana. Dr. Edgar Johnwick, the director of the leprosy hospital, sat entranced as Brand described the program at Karigiri. His American competitive instincts were stirred. "It's quite apparent your patients in India get a better rehabilitation program than our patients in the U.S.," he said with obvious concern. "As an officer of the U.S. Public Health Service, I can't accept that. Would you consider coming here and setting up a similar program?"

The Brands, British subjects who had served in India, were reluctant to introduce yet a third culture into their children's lives. But Johnwick proved to be the consummate salesman. He promised that the USPHS would fully support all of Brand's consulting work overseas, and that Carville would create a position in ophthalmology for his wife. "It's the least we can do," Johnwick said, after a few phone calls to Washington for authorization.

Carville had never had a full-time ophthalmologist on the staff and the administration was offering Margaret Brand a position which existed almost nowhere else in the world. This new offer would give her the opportunity to be involved in

Leprosy in the U.S.— The Carville Story

Carville was established as a state leprosy hospital in 1894 by the Board of Control for the Louisiana Leper Home to care for seven patients who were housed in New Orleans under very poor conditions. Dr. Isadore Dyer referred to it as the "pest house." The first leprosy patients were taken to Carville at night by barge and unloaded on the banks of the Mississippi River near the small town of Carville. Shelter was provided in what had been a working plantation, leased from the absentee landowners by the State of Louisiana.

In 1896, the Catholic order, The Daughters of Charity of the St. Vincent's de Paul, began supplying staff to the hospital, and continued to do so for the next one hundred years. In 1921, the facility was taken over by the United States government and became part of the Marine Hospital system and the U.S. Public Health Service. Today the Federal Bureau of Primary Health Care still administers the U.S. national leprosy program.

The Carville facility was first known as the Louisiana Leper Home. There have been a number of name changes, including at one time, the Gillis W. Long Hansen's Disease Center. Currently it is known as the National Hansen's Disease Program. Mostly it was known simply as Carville, named after the small town and post office about two miles from the hospital. Until the 1950s, public health laws mandated that newly diagnosed leprosy cases in the U.S. must be taken to Carville for treatment. At its peak there were about 415 residents.

Over time, Carville developed into a self-contained village, with a well-equipped hospital staffed by resident physicians, small shops, a school, a library, a barbershop, and recreational facilities. This isolation was by design, since patients were not allowed to leave the premises until they were declared noninfectious. As a consequence, many persons, including younger persons, spent most of their lives at Carville. This policy was relaxed in the 1960s.

Carville became an internationally recognized center for leprosy diagnosis, treatment, training, and research, both clinical and laboratory. A major breakthrough occured in 1941, when under the direction of Dr. Guy Faget, a sulfone drug— promin—proved to be the first drug effective in the treatment for leprosy. From this early work, another sulfone, commonly known as dapsone, was developed. This drug in combination with rifampin and clofazimine became the miracle cure for which the world had been waiting. By the 1950s, patients were regularly being cured.

Another major breakthrough occurred in 1970 when Carville laboratory workers discovered that wild armadillos, plentiful in Louisiana and neighboring states, carry the bacteria that causes leprosy. This was significant because armadillos housed in captivity provided a source of bacteria for laboratory research. Until then, bacteria could not be grown in laboratories and this hindered further research. Even today the bacteria cannot be grown in artificial laboratory media.

American Leprosy Missions has had a long and mutually valued association with Carville. In 1928, ALM contributed funds for a Protestant chapel. ALM's Dr. Felton Ross conducted a series of one-week training courses at Carville in the 1970s and 1980s for medical missionaries who were planning to work overseas with leprosy. Though initially in great demand, these courses were eventually phased out as programs were shifted to the countries where leprosy was endemic.

A number of Carville staff also served on the ALM Board of Directors. Included were Dr. John Trautman, director of the center from 1968 to 1988; Emanuel Faria, the longtime editor of the Star magazine; Dr. Leo Yoder, physician and chief of medicine from 1982 to 1997; Dr. Margaret Brand, chief of ophthalmology; and Dr. Paul Brand, chief of the rehabilitation branch. ALM has continued to fund special projects including educational materials and laboratory research projects.

Carville patients have been active in addressing the problem of stigma, including advocacy to substitute the name Hansen's disease for leprosy. The Star magazine began publication in 1941, with some well-known patients such as Stanley Stein and Emanuel Faria serving as editors. A number of books have been written by patients such as *Alone No Longer* by Stanley Stein and *Miracle at Carville*

by Betty Martin. Betty Martin was one of the first patients to receive sulfone drugs in 1941 and was eventually cured of the disease.

As patient numbers decreased and treatment was provided in Public Health Service clinics in the U.S., the Carville facility became cost ineffective. In 1999 it was returned to the State of Louisiana and the Louisiana National Guard as a training center for at-risk youth. The National Hansen's Disease Programs were moved to Baton Rouge, where some fifty older disabled patients are cared for. It also serves as a referral center for complicated cases. By their choice, about twenty patients continued to reside at the Carville site. The former Carville staff dining hall has been converted into the National Hansen's Disease Museum. It is open to visitors daily during business hours. The laboratory research branch continues as a significant research center in facilities leased from the Louisiana State University School of Veterinary Medicine in Baton Rouge.

Currently, there are approximately seven thousand patients on the U.S. leprosy registry (that includes all patients since the registry began). In 2002 and 2003, there were 113 and 130 new cases reported respectively. The majority of these are from first generation immigrants to the U.S., although a small number of cases continue to occur in the U.S.-born persons.

—**Dr. Leo Yoder**

ocular leprosy on a daily basis—the very position she had recently given up at Karigiri. The salaries for the Brands would allow them to afford transporting their children in England back to Carville without worry during holidays so that those attending boarding school in England could continue their course work.

The Brands came to the United States at a propitious time for scientific research. The government generously funded medical programs even when, as in the case of leprosy, they primarily benefited people elsewhere. (The registered leprosy population in the United States numbered only about six thousand.) Carville had nearly as many staff members as patients and the Brands were able to obtain research equipment that would have seemed lavish in India. For example, Paul Brand soon learned of an exciting technology, thermography, which showed promise for medical applications, and ordered a forty-thousand-dollar machine for their clinic. The thermograph was an elaborate mechanism for measuring temperature.

In India he had recognized the importance of monitoring the temperature of patients' feet and hands. Insensitive to pain, they do not usually know if they have damaged tissue beneath the surface, but the body responds anyway by rushing an increased blood supply to the damaged area. A spot of infection in the foot, for instance, requires three to four times the normal blood supply in order to heal the wound and control the infection. Brand had trained his hands to detect these "hot spots," practicing so that eventually he learned to perceive a change in temperature as small as one-and-a-half degrees Celsius and sometimes even one-and-a-quarter degrees. If he felt a warm spot on a patient's foot, he knew that it probably meant inflammation and thus kept a careful eye on it. If the high temperature persisted, he would take an X-ray to see if the underlying bone had cracked.

Now, on the thermogram monitor or on a printout, he could see an entire foot at once, displaying variances in temperature as small as one-quarter of a degree. Cool areas of the skin showed up as green or blue; warmer areas appeared violet, orange or red; the hottest areas glowed yellow or white. The thermograph was fascinating and fun to operate because it produced such colorful maps of the hand or foot. He experimented with the machine for several months before realizing its true potential: the thermograph's remarkable precision allowed him to detect problems at such an early stage that it functioned essentially as a time-delayed pain system.

In India, Brand had learned to contain the damage by aggressively treating visible injuries—blisters, cuts, punctures—right away. Far more difficult was the damage caused by pressure sores: these developed under the surface and only broke open into an ulcer at a later stage. The thermograph offered, for the first time, the ability to peer under the skin and observe such inflammation before it exposed itself on the skin surface. Now medical staff could actually *prevent* ulcers by arresting tissue breakdown sooner.

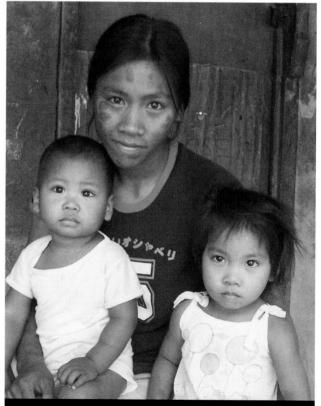

Even after a patient is no longer contagious, a condition called "Leprosy Reaction" can cause disfiguring spots and nodules.

If the thermograph revealed a warm spot on a hand or foot, therapists could immobilize the limb for a few days, or at least reduce weight bearing, to keep the patient from further harm and heal the commencing problem. Compared to a healthy pain system, of course, the high-tech thermograph was rather crude, for it detected a problem after the fact, not before. (The beauty of pain is that it lets you know right away when you are hurting yourself.) Nevertheless, it gave new precision in monitoring potential problems. Brand began requiring Carville patients to come for regular hand-and-foot checkups with the thermograph.

~~~

He faced initial resistance from the Patients' Federation, whose officers objected to any screening that might threaten patients' jobs. For example, one of the early screenings revealed a hot spot of inflammation on a patient's thumb. After questioning him, Brand learned that his job included the task of raking up grass behind a mower. "You must stop that for a time, until this inflammation settles down," the doctor advised him. He promptly reported the conversation to the Patients' Federation. Neither he nor the federation could understand why a doctor was concerned about a thumb that did not appear to be injured and did not hurt.

In time, however, the thermograph proved itself. The Carville clinic worked with the Patients' Federation in finding substitute jobs for endangered patients, and the hospital began seeing a marked reduction in ulcers and chronic infections. The investment in the machine paid for itself many times over.

Cries and Whispers

Thanks to generous government grants, Paul Brand hired nine additional staff members in the rehabilitation department at Carville. Working as a team, engineers, scientists, computer experts, and biologists thoroughly investigated all aspects of the hazards produced by insensitivity to pain. In most cases, as with the thermograph, they were not breaking new ground, but rather adding sophistication and precision to the principles first learned in India.

Gradually, a new understanding of how pain protects normal limbs emerged, and at the same time the Brands began to view painlessness as one of the greatest curses that can befall a human being. In India they had relied mainly on visual cues—blisters from a lamp, rat bites—whereas in Carville the tools at their disposal allowed them to solve the more obscure mysteries of tissue breakdown. They gained an ever-increasing sense of awe and gratitude for the extraordinary ways in which pain daily protects every healthy person.

Research confirmed there are at least three basic ways in which danger constantly presents itself to a pain-insensitive person.

1) Direct Injury

Many direct injuries encountered at Carville were familiar, for they had been tracked extensively at Vellore. The fingers of smokers often displayed the pattern of "kissing wounds," and the fingers of cooks were betrayed by burns from cooking pots. Some direct injuries at Carville were new. In one case that Margaret Brand treated, a woman named Eva hurt herself by using mascara. Characteristically, she had lost her eyebrows and eyelashes because of leprosy bacilli invasion. Each day she painted mascara on both areas with a brush, but because her hands and eyes were insensitive she often missed the eyelid margin and stabbed the pigment into her eye. Brand warned her strongly that she would soon damage her eye irreversibly. Eva ignored all these admonitions, and one day she explained why. "You don't understand," she said, "it's more important how the world sees me than how I see the world."

As a hand surgeon, Brand was called upon to treat a steady procession of direct injuries. The typical person suffers one minor wound a week, or about four thousand in a lifetime. The fingers and thumbs account for 95 percent of these wounds: paper cuts, cigarette burns, thorns, splinters. Leprosy patients, without the safeguard of pain, experience wounds much more frequently, and because they keep on using the affected hand, severe damage often results. At least 90 percent of the insensitive hands examined by leprosy specialists show scars and signs of deformity or injury.

Direct injuries were by far the easiest to deal with. Patients understood them because they could see the damage. Brand merely had to keep the finger in a splint until it healed and then, just as he had done in India, teach patients the need for constant vigilance. He urged them to take responsibility for parts of their bodies they could not feel, relying on other senses for their clues. "Test your bath water with a thermometer in advance," he cautioned. "And never grip the handle of a tool without looking first to see if there's an edge that might cut you, or a splinter to stick into you." Posters went up in the hospital, graphically illustrating the most common hazards.

The incidence of direct injuries at Carville began to decrease, especially as they relied on tools like the thermograph to monitor the early problems under the skin. Just as important, the patients improved at caring for wounds after an injury. A foot wound will heal if a patient tends to it. If, however, the patient keeps walking on the injured foot, infection may set in and spread through the foot, destroying bones and joints, and amputation becomes inevitable. In the six years prior to a campaign against injuries, twenty-seven amputations had been performed at Carville; over the next few years the rate fell to zero.

2) Constant Stress

Other damage was much harder to track down. Human skin is tough: normally, it takes more than five hundred pounds of pressure per square inch to penetrate the skin and cause injury. But a constant, unrelieved pressure as low as one pound per square inch can do damage.

Press a glass slide against your fingertip and the skin will blanch. Hold it there for a few hours and the skin, deprived of blood supply, will die.

Brand learned much about constant stress from a friendly pig named Sherman, who made an ideal subject for experiments because pigskin has properties similar to human skin. The researchers would anesthetize Sherman, put him in a plaster half-cast to keep him still, and apply very slight pressure to designated spots on his back. A cylindrical piston kept the pressure at a constant one pound per square inch for five to seven hours. Subsequent thermograms clearly showed that this very slight pressure caused inflammation in and under the skin. The pressure spot turned red, and hair permanently stopped growing there. If they had kept up the pressure longer, an ulcer would have developed on Sherman's back.

The pressure spots on Sherman's back illustrate the process behind bedsores, the bane of modern hospitals. Some bedsores are as horrible as any surface wound you might find in a battlefield hospital. All bedsores trace back to the same cause: constant stress. A paralyzed or insensitive person tends to lie on the same spot hour after hour, shutting off the blood supply, and after about four hours of unrelieved pressure the tissue begins to die. People with a well-functioning nervous system do not get bedsores. A steady stream of quiet messages from the pain network will keep an active body tossing and turning in bed, redistributing the stress among the body's cells. If these quiet messages are ignored, the distressed region sends out a louder cry of real pain that forces the person to shift a buttock or turn over on one side, thus relieving the pressure.

Findings about constant stress helped Brand and his Carville team understand why a leprosy patient has such difficulty fitting shoes. He was surprised to find that U.S. patients had about the same incidence of amputated feet as their counterparts in India, many of whom went barefoot. The problem, he discovered, was that they were wearing shoes designed for patients who can feel pain. The risk of constant stress from poorly designed shoes is every bit as dangerous as the risk of direct injury from going barefoot. If a pain-sensitive person's shoes feel too tight, he or she removes them. The leprosy patient, who feels no pain, leaves a tight shoe on even after pressure has shut off the blood supply. Carville therapists began to require patients to change shoes twice in a day, at least once every five hours—a simple measure that, if followed, prevents ulcers from ischemic pressure.

The thermograph detects problems, but addressing those problems requires the cooperation of patients. Paul Brand remembered his first thermograph session with José, a "certified negative" patient who came from California for monitoring once every six months. José's toes had shrunken due to bone resorption, and pressure sores kept the infection from clearing up. Yet he stubbornly refused to wear orthopedic shoes. "They're too ugly," he said. José had a clean, unmarked face and no one suspected him of being a leprosy patient. "I have a good job selling furniture. If I wear the ugly shoes, someone may guess I have a disease. And then I will lose my job."

Brand had high hopes that the thermograph might persuade José to swallow his pride. He had never taken the staff's warnings very seriously because his feet looked fine on the surface. Now Brand could show José on a thermogram exactly where the inflammation was developing. "Look at the hot white spot on your smallest toe. Do you see where your narrow shoe is pressing too tight?" José nodded, and Brand felt encouraged.

"You can't see anything yet, and you don't feel pain. But that white color is a severe danger sign of problems under the surface. You'll have an ulcer there very soon." He used a stern tone of voice. "José, mark my words, you may lose that toe if you don't do something."

José listened politely, but still refused to wear the therapeutic shoes. "Well then," the doctor said, "go shopping for some new shoes that you like. Buy the next largest size, and let me build

up around the pressure points with a soft padding that will spread out the stress." He agreed to this plan, but when he left Carville, Brand had no confidence that José would actually wear the new shoes.

Sure enough, six months later José returned with an open ulcer on his small toe. The toe had visibly shrunk, and X-rays revealed progressive bone absorption from the chronic infection. José received this news with nonchalance. Because his feet did not hurt him, he ignored them. Nothing the doctor said convinced him to care. During the next few years Paul watched with a feeling of total helplessness as José let other bones in his toes get absorbed. He ended up with two severely shortened stumps with little bumps where his toes had been, solely because he refused to wear less-than-stylish shoes. The thermograph could give a visual warning, yes, but one which lacked the compulsion of pain.

It took the Vellore staff years of baffling research to comprehend fully a basic fact of human anatomy: any gentle stress repeatedly applied to the same spot can destroy living tissue. One clap of a hand does no damage; a thousand consecutive claps may cause pain and real damage. In walking, the mechanical force of the thousandth step is no greater than that of the first step, but foot tissue is vulnerable to the cumulative impact of force. The foot's main enemy turned out to be not thorns and nails, but the normal, everyday stresses of walking.

Every healthy person knows something of this phenomenon. You buy a new pair of shoes, put them on, and start walking around the house and yard. For the first few hours they feel fine, yet after a while the stiff leather begins to wear on your little toe and a rough edge grates against your heel. Instinctively you limp, shortening your stride and redistributing the stress to other parts of the foot. Ignore the warning signals, and a blister will pop up and soon you experience acute pain. At that point, you probably remove the new shoes and put on some soft slippers for relief. On average it takes about a week to break in new shoes, a process that involves adaptations both in the leather of the shoe and the leather of your foot. The shoe gets softer and more compliant to your foot's shape, while your foot grows extra layers of callus for protection at the stress points.

This entire process is foreign to a leprosy patient. Because he feels no pain from his little toe and heel, his stride never adjusts. After a blister rises, he still keeps walking, oblivious. The blister bursts, and an ulcer begins to form. Even so, he puts the shoes back on the next day, and the next, each time damaging more tissue. Infection may set in. If it goes untreated, that hot infection may spread into the bone, where it will not heal unless it gets complete rest. Tiny pieces of bone fragment break off until eventually the infection leads to the loss of toes or even the entire foot. All this time, the leprosy patient may continue to walk on the injury site, showing not the slightest sign of a limp.

The results of Paul Brand's research on the dangers of painlessness had a dramatic effect on the treatment of leprosy and other anesthetic diseases worldwide. Fifteen million victims of leprosy gained hope that, with proper care, they could preserve their toes and fingers and eyesight. Later, he applied the same principles to the insensitive feet of diabetics, helping to prevent, by one estimate, seventy thousand amputations annually in the United States alone.

3) Repetitive Stress

In retrospect, the most valuable product of Paul Brand's two decades of pain research was new insight into how ordinary, "harmless" stresses can cause severe damage to skin if they are repeated thousands of times. He first became aware of this syndrome in India while testing different kinds of footwear, but the research labs at Carville provided the tools to discern exactly how repetitive stress does its work.

For several decades he had puzzled over why the simple act of walking represented such a threat to a leprosy patient. How is it, he wondered, that a healthy person can walk ten miles without injury while a leprosy patient often cannot? In an attempt to answer this question, Carville engineers rigged up a repetitive stress machine that reproduced the stresses of walking or running. The machine's tiny mechanical hammer repeatedly strikes the same area with a force calibrated to what a small region of the foot may endure while walking.

Researchers used laboratory rats for these experiments, putting them to sleep and strapping one footpad to the machine which proceeded to tap their footpads with a steady, rhythmic force. While the rats slept, their feet went for a simulated run. The results proved conclusively that a "harmless" force, repeated often enough, does indeed cause tissue breakdown. If researchers gave the rats enough rest between runs, they could build up layers of callus; if not, they could trace the stages of inflammation that would result in an open sore.

Several times Brand tested the machine on his own fingers. The first day he put his finger under the hammer, he felt no pain up to about one thousand strokes. The sensation felt rather pleasant, like a vibro-massage. After one thousand strokes, though, he began to feel tenderness. The second day it took far fewer strokes of the tiny hammer for him to sense tenderness. On the third day, he felt acute pain almost immediately.

He now knew that tiny pressures, if repeated often enough, could damage tissue, so that under certain circumstances the ordinary act of walking might indeed prove dangerous. Yet he still had not answered the underlying question: What made the feet of leprosy patients more vulnerable to repetitive stress? He could walk ten miles without injury; why couldn't they?

Another invention, the slipper-sock, helped solve that mystery. Brand hired a chemical research company to develop a tiny micro-capsule that would break down due to pressure. After many false starts he ended up with a slipper-sock made up of a thin foam that incorporated thousands of micro-capsules of hard wax. The capsules contained a dye that turns blue in an alkaline medium. It took quite a lot of force to break the capsules, but the wax—exactly like human skin—would also break when subjected to the repetitive stress of many small forces. Now he had a convenient way to measure the pressure points involved in walking.

Volunteer staff put on these socks under their shoes and started walking. After they had gone a few paces they removed the shoes and noted the highest pressure points, which were the first spots to turn blue. As they walked farther, the blue areas spread wider, and the initial pressure points deepened in color. After fifty paces or so the slipper-sock gave a good picture of all the danger areas. Then Brand tried the slipper-socks on patients. After poring over thousands of used slipper-socks, he learned a lot about walking, but nothing more important than this: a person with an insensitive foot never changes his stride. In contrast, a healthy person changes his stride constantly.

A physical therapist in the hospital volunteered to run eight miles around the cement floor corridors of the Carville hospital in his stocking feet, pausing every two miles to let Brand take thermographic readings and test his stride in a slipper-sock. The first slipper-sock impression showed his normal walking pattern, a long stride with a high lift and a push off the great toe. The thermogram taken after two miles revealed a hot spot on his overworked great toe, and the slipper-sock showed that the main pressure point had moved to the inner side of his sole. After four miles, the signs of pressure shifted as his stride spontaneously adjusted. Now the outside of his foot was outlined in bright blue, showing that his weight had shifted to the outside, away from the great toe, as the inner side took a long rest. By the time he ran the last two miles both the thermogram and the slipper-sock confirmed that he had again changed the way he put his feet to the ground: now the outer edge of his foot was getting hot and breaking the microcapsules.

The full set of thermograms and slipper-socks revealed a startling phenomenon: taken together, the socks portrayed a complete map of his foot, with strong blue dye at many different points. While the therapist himself was concentrating on jogging, his foot was sending out subconscious messages of pain. Although these tiny whispers from individual pressure and pain cells never made it all the way to his conscious brain, they did make it to his spinal cord and lower brain, which ordered subtle adjustments in his stride. Over the course of his run, the foot distributed pressure evenly, keeping any one spot from receiving too much repetitive stress.

Brand never sent a leprosy patient on an eight-mile run, for that would be totally irresponsible. The reason shows up vividly in slipper-socks taken from a patient's shorter runs:

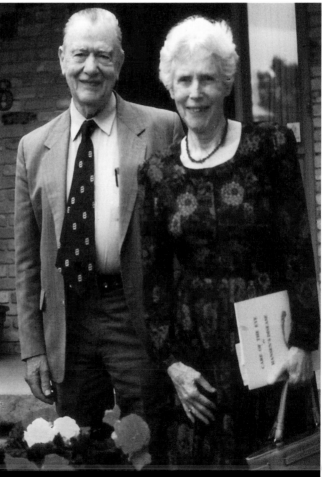

Drs. Paul and Margaret Brand in the late 1980s (photo by Frank Duerksen)

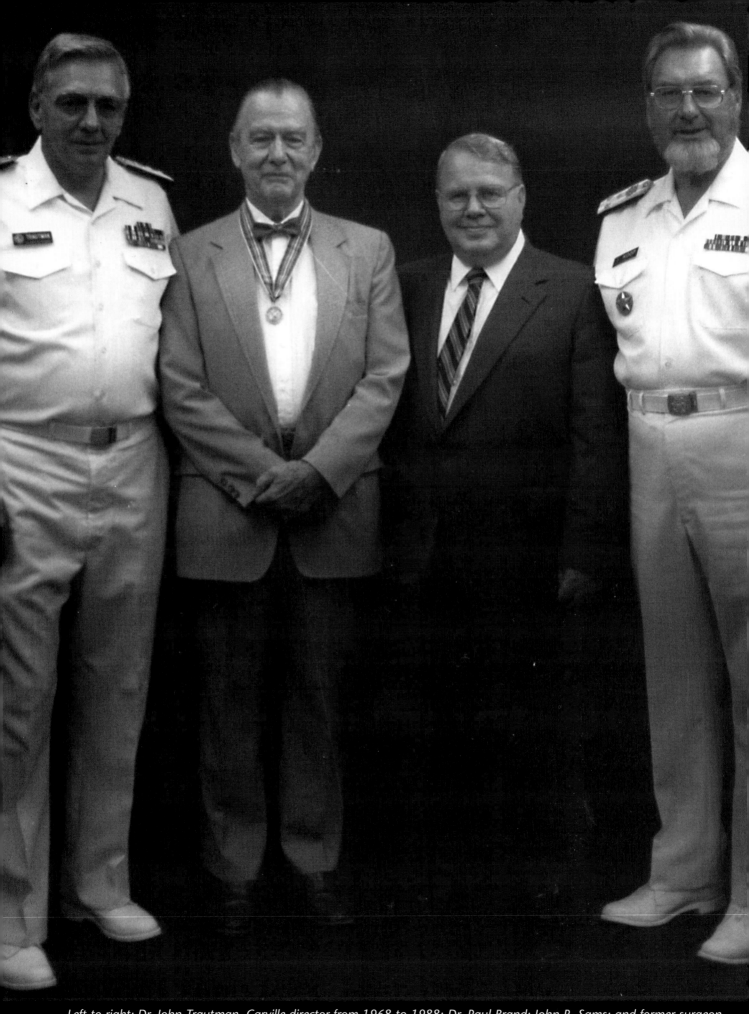

Left to right: Dr. John Trautman, Carville director from 1968 to 1988; Dr. Paul Brand; John R. Sams; and former surgeon general of the United States, Dr. C. Everett Koop

impressions before and after the run were virtually identical. The leprosy patient's stride never changed. Its pain pathways silenced, the central nervous system never perceived a need to make adjustments, and so the same pressure—ten, twenty, or even sixty pounds per square inch—kept pounding on the same square inches of foot surface. If Brand had sent a leprosy patient on an eight-mile run, he would have gotten a thermogram with just one or two areas of angry hot spots, the signs of damaged tissue. A few days later, he would likely see a plantar ulcer on the sole of the foot. Healthy long-distance runners seldom get plantar ulcers; leprosy patients often do.

A healthy person can sense the rising danger from constant stress. At first the finger or toe feels perfectly comfortable. After perhaps an hour a feeling of irritation sets in, followed by mild pain. Finally, intolerable pain intervenes just before the point of real damage. Paul Brand noted:

> I can observe this cycle at work whenever I attend a banquet. The culprit is fashion: when women dress for special occasions they fall under the evil spell of shoe designers who favor narrow, pointed shoes and high heels. I glance under the table after an hour or two of dinner and speeches and observe that half the women have kicked off their fashionable shoes; they are giving their feet a few minutes of unimpeded circulation before subjecting them to another round of bloodlessness.

> I notice a similar pattern whenever I deliver a lecture. As long as I manage to hold the audience's attention, I see much less restless activity. They are consciously attending to what I am saying, and thus squelching or ignoring the subtle messages of discomfort. But as soon as my lecture gets boring, their mental concentration wanders and instinctively they tune in to the faint messages of distress from cells that have been sat on for too long. I can judge the effectiveness of my

speech by watching how frequently members of the audience cross and uncross their legs and shift about in their seats.

Nowadays, repetitive stress injuries are widely recognized as a major problem in high-technology environments. Almost two hundred thousand U.S. office and factory workers each year are treated for such conditions, accounting for more than half of the country's occupational illnesses. The frequency has doubled in less than a decade, mainly because technology tends to reduce the variety of movements required and thus increase repetitive stress. For example, so innocuous an action as typing or operating a video game joystick, can by constant repetition subject the wrist to pressures that produce carpal tunnel syndrome. Computer keyboards are far more likely to cause injury than mechanical typewriters because the typist no longer has the relief of reaching up to move the carriage or pausing to change the paper. In the U.S., repetitive stress injuries currently cost about seven billion dollars a year in lost productivity and medical costs.

Legacy

Paul Brand spent two decades at the leprosy hospital in Carville, retiring in 1986 at the age of seventy-two. His wife, Margaret, retired the next year at the age of sixty-eight. Shortly afterward they moved to a small cottage overlooking Puget Sound in Seattle. Brand served a few terms as president of the International Christian Medical and Dental Society; he consulted with the World Health Organization; and into his eighties continued to lecture throughout the world. His work on reconstruction of leprosy hands and feet won him awards and acclaim: hand-surgery procedures named in his honor, two Hunterian Lectures, the prestigious Albert Lasker Award, an appointment as commander of the Order of the British Empire by Queen Elizabeth II, and selection as the only Westerner to serve on the Mahatma Gandhi Foundation.

Margaret Brand, who had initially begged for any medical specialty "as long as it isn't in eyes," and who had never formally qualified as an ophthalmologist, became one of the world's foremost experts on the ocular problems of leprosy. She made presentations at the International Leprosy Congress, and well into her eighties she continued to give annual clinics at the hospital in Karigiri. She also served several terms on the board of the American Leprosy Missions.

In his twilight years, Paul Brand accepted many invitations from medical schools that asked him to address the dehumanization of medicine. Today, high-tech medicine, HMO insurance policies, and increasing specialization conspire to squelch the very instincts that draw many of the best students into the field. Brand expresses the guiding principle of his medical career this way: "The most precious possession any human being has is his spirit—his will to live, his sense of dignity, his personality. Though technically we may be concerned with tendons, bones, and nerve endings, we must never lose sight of the *person* we are treating."

It takes a few pennies a day to arrest leprosy's progress with sulfone drugs. It takes thousands of dollars, and the painstaking care of skilled professionals, to restore to wholeness a patient in whom the disease has spread unchecked. The surgeries and rehabilitation pioneered by Paul and Margaret Brand stretched over months and sometimes years, involving hands and feet, eyes, and repairs to the face. Both doctors lobbied hard against any agency pronouncing a leprosy patient "cured" by one standard alone, the lack of active bacilli.

Paul Brand once mused on why there are Christian missions devoted exclusively to leprosy. Much of the Brands's work in India was funded by The Leprosy Mission of England, sister organization to American Leprosy Missions. "I know of no Arthritis Mission or Diabetes Mission," he said. "The answer, I think, relates to the incredible stigma that has surrounded leprosy for so many centuries. To work with leprosy required more than a natural instinct of compassion; it required a kind of supernatural calling. People such as Father Damien, who ministered to leprosy patients in Hawaii and then contracted the disease himself, believed that human beings, no matter what their affliction, should never be cast aside. It was up to the church to care for the sick, the unwanted, the unloved."

He then mentioned a comment made by Mother Teresa as he consulted with her on a leprosy clinic she was opening in Calcutta. "We have drugs for people with diseases like leprosy," she said. "But these drugs do not treat the main problem, the disease of being unwanted. That's what my sisters hope to provide."

Dr. Paul Brand passed away in July 2003 at the age of eighty-nine. In the leprosy world he was renowned for his pioneer work in hand surgery. In the Christian world, he was celebrated for his wonderful writing and spiritual insights. To friends, family, and colleagues, and patients he was a giver of dignity; an enabler, and a healer. The man who learned carpentry before he studied medicine planted his feet firmly in the footsteps of another carpenter and walked beside the people he treated. He did not walk ahead. He did not turn away. He touched people who hurt and used his gifts to restore them in body and spirit.

Margaret Brand continues to live in Seattle and consults on leprosy ophthalmology in other countries. Their stories are told in three books: *Fearfully and Wonderfully Made, In His Image*, and *The Gift of Pain*, from which much of the material in this chapter was adapted.

ABOUT THE AUTHOR

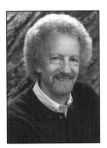

*P*hilip Yancey *earned graduate degrees in communications and English from Wheaton College Graduate School and the University of Chicago. He joined the staff of* Campus Life *magazine in 1971, and worked there as editor for eight years.*

Since 1978, Yancey has primarily concentrated on writing. More than six hundred of his articles have appeared in eighty different publications, including Reader's Digest, Publishers Weekly, National Wildlife, Saturday Evening Post, Christian Century, *and* The Reformed Journal. *He writes articles and a monthly column for* Christianity Today *magazine, which he serves as editor-at-large. He also serves as cochair of the Editorial Board for Books and Culture, a recent publication of* Christianity Today.

Yancey's sixteen books include Where Is God When it Hurts?, The Student Bible, *and* Disappointment with God. *These books have won eleven Gold Medallion Awards from the Evangelical Christian Publishers Association and have sold more than five million copies. Other titles,* Fearfully and Wonderfully Made, In His Image, *and* The Gift of Pain, *were coauthored with Dr. Paul Brand. Christian bookstore managers selected* The Jesus I Never Knew *as the 1996 Book of the Year, and* What's So Amazing About Grace? *won the same award in 1998. His most recent books are* The Bible Jesus Read, Reaching for the Invisible God, Soul Survivor, *and* Rumors of Another World.

The Yanceys lived in downtown Chicago for many years before moving to a very different environment in Colorado. They enjoy hiking, wildlife, and all the other delights of the Rocky Mountains.

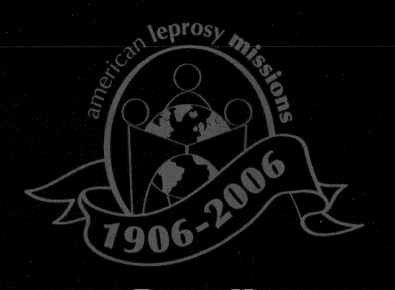

Part II

Chapter 6

ALM News Throughout the Century

by Eugene Wilson

1911—William M. Danner Appointed First Full-Time Secretary

1911

Attracted to leave a promising career with the Kellogg Company to join a fledgling mission focused on a cause the world wanted to ignore, Danner led the board in making a series of decisions that were breathtaking in scope. The newly appointed secretary was authorized to organize a publicity campaign, recruit a board of reference, solicit the involvement of young people's societies, begin a mail solicitation campaign, and increase participation in interdenominational gatherings.

The board also appointed two field secretaries and authorized increased contact with denominational mission boards and laymen's committees. Public presentations were well received, but contributions were meager. Under Danner's visionary leadership the number of auxiliaries and local committees in the U.S. increased to thirty-two.

In 1915 Danner led the board in advocating for the establishment of a national leprosarium in the U.S. The obstacles were immense. First the bill had to be passed by Congress. Then more than fifty sites were explored, but most later withdrew because of local "not-in-my-backyard" objections. The bill was finally passed in 1917. Writing to Danner almost twenty-five years later, Dr. George McCoy, the longtime head of the National Institutes of Health said, "The splendid Federal Leprosarium at Carville is a monument to you and you alone."

In 1937, due to ill health, Danner resigned from the work to which he had become deeply attached and with which he had been closely associated for twenty-six tumultuous years.

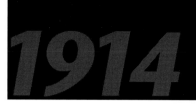

1914—Protestant Chapel Built at Carville

The first Protestant worship service at Carville was held January 21, 1914. The minister was Dr. Theodore Hahn from New Orleans, whose father had served the needs of leprosy patients in India. With Danner's encouragement, Hahn and area ministers conducted services, eventually leading to the construction of a Protestant chapel with funds raised by the ALM.

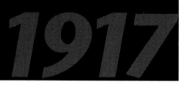

1917—American Mission to Lepers

American Mission to Lepers was officially incorporated in the State of New York on July 31, 1917, a natural sequence of maturity and necessity. The original article in the certificate of incorporation reads as follows:

> That the principal objectives for which the proposed Corporation is to be formed are generally to preach the gospel to those suffering from leprosy and to aid them through the relief of their sufferings and supply their wants.

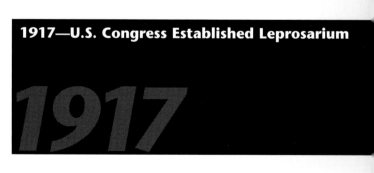

1917—U.S. Congress Established Leprosarium

The surgeon general of USPHS was ordered to prepare rules and regulations for patients to be admitted. Though a great victory, implementation of the bill was a long struggle, due to difficulty in finding an acceptable site. The national leprosarium actually opened on February 1, 1921.

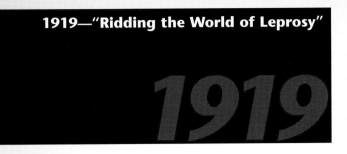

1919—"Ridding the World of Leprosy"

This was the bold headline assigned to the prophetic action taken by the American committee in 1919. Though it proved to be premature, it aroused international excitement. The resolution read as follows:

> . . . that we re-affirm our convictions that the purpose of the Mission to Lepers includes not only the evangelization and amelioration of their physical condition and the supplying of their simple, natural wants but also a comprehensive program to "Rid the World of Leprosy."

A few weeks later the secretary was authorized to publish a sixty-four-page booklet entitled "Ridding the World of Leprosy" to be sold "for an amount not to exceed 15 cents." Five thousand copies were to be prepared at once and type was kept standing until further orders.

The booklet attracted the attention of health officials in Washington, D.C., who summoned Secretary Danner to a meeting sponsored by the predecessor to what is known today as the Pan American Health Organization. A Spanish translation of the booklet was authorized and distributed throughout the southern hemisphere.

1921—The Vision Spread Beyond Asia

In October 1921 the board received the survey of South American lepers provided by the Commonwealth Fund and authorized participation in a conference to discuss leprosy in South America.

In May 1922, the board heard the report of Dr. W. H. Hudnut's visit to a leper colony in Cameroon, Africa. He also visited the Presbyterian mission station and the hospital at Elat, where he "preached for the lepers and conducted a sacramental service." He saw lepers everywhere, emphasizing the great need of some special survey in Africa.

1921—A Board of Reference Appointed

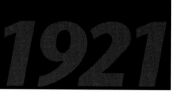

The American Committee appointed a Board of Reference to gain viability. This included some of the best-known churchmen and mission executives of the time, including the following:

- William Jennings Bryan, later invited to become vice president of the society. (No reply is recorded.)

- Dr. George W. McCoy, surgeon, U.S. Public Health Service, Island of Molokai, Hawaii, author of the bill establishing a national leprosarium in the United States.

- Dr. Isadore Dyer, Dean, Tulane School of Medicine, Louisiana, said to "know more about leprosy in Louisiana, and probably in the United States, than any other physician."

- Dr. Victor G. Heiser, Philippine leprologist who addressed the Sixty-fourth U.S. Congress hearings to examine the problem of leprosy in the United States and the need for a national leprosarium.

1926—Chinese Mission to Lepers Organized

During the general secretary's visit to China in 1926, he helped to organize the Chinese Mission to Lepers. The Rev. T. C. Wu, a young Baptist minister educated in America, was selected as secretary. With American Mission support, the Chinese Mission established four hospitals and a score of skin clinics before the country was disrupted by the war with Japan.

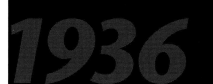

Dr. Emory Ross was appointed general secretary in 1936, upon the resignation of William Danner due to failing health, with extreme regret and gratitude. Ross, sometimes known as a "little Schweitzer," had served thirty-five years in Africa. He was also secretary of the Congo Christian Council. His report identified three key relationships for ALM:

I. The American Public which supports it.
II. The church organizations through which it works.
III. The governments, and increased cooperation with them.

1939—Kellersberger Became General Secretary

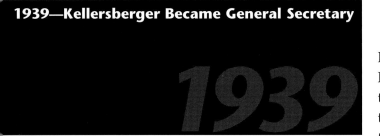

Early in 1939 Dr. and Mrs. Eugene Kellersberger felt led to close the African chapter of their missionary career after almost twenty-five years. Dr. Kellersberger was one of the best-known physicians in Central Africa; he also served as secretary of the medical committee of the Protestant Council and was superintendent of the leper colony of the Presbyterian Church (South) at Biganga, Congo. Belgium's King Leopold made him a member of the Royal Commission for the protection of natives. The ALM Board invited them to continue their service subject to the approval of the Foreign Missions Committee of the Presbyterian Church.

1941—Results of Promin

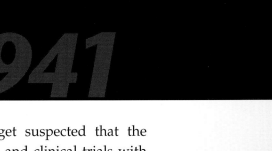

The American Mission to Lepers took great satisfaction in publishing the results of the use of the sulfone family of drugs on patients who had volunteered for the painful and dangerous experiment since 1941. First used by Dr. G. H. Faget, Medical Director at Carville, Promin was a derivative of diamino-diphenylsulfone (DDS). Dr. Faget suspected that the diamino-diphenylsulfone content was the active principle, and clinical trials with dapsone (DDS) confirmed his suspicions. This not only opened the chemotherapeutic era in treating leprosy, but raised again the prospect of a cure.

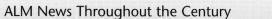

1950—Name Change

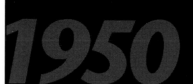

After prolonged and sometimes heated debate, the Board of Directors agreed that effective January 1, 1949: "The name of this Corporation is American Leprosy Missions, Incorporated."

1950—New York Academy of Sciences Held Two-Day Symposium on Hansen's Disease

Dr. Eugene R. Kellersberger, who for years fought the unwarranted social stigma attached to so-called leprosy, delivered a challenging paper on the status of leprosy treatment.

1951—Gene Phillips Clemes Began Twenty-Six-Year Association with ALM

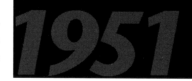

Gene Phillips Clemes joined the staff of the American Leprosy Missions on May 14, 1951 as director of public relations, a newly created position. Her writing skills and public relations skills were directed toward promotion. She collaborated with Dr. Emory Ross in writing the book, *New Hearts, New Faces*, published in 1954 by Friendship Press. A second book, *Drum Call of Hope*, by Gene Phillips was published and widely distributed in 1960.

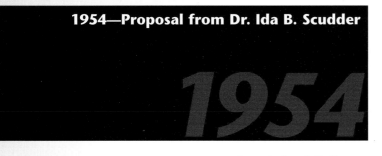

1954—Proposal from Dr. Ida B. Scudder

Dr. Ida B. Scudder and Vellore Christian Medical College proposed an expenditure of $75,000 for the development of leprosy work. "Dr. Ida" had initiated roadside clinics for the treatment of leprosy even as the Medical College was developing. ALM's postwar plan stated in "Against a Worldwide Enemy":

> In Vellore, center of the highest incidence of the disease, the American Mission to Lepers will build a training center, including a 200-patient sanatorium in the All India Medical College, the magnificent modern institution now being erected on initial foundations long since laid with the cooperation of 25 denominations. Dr. Robert Cochrane, leprologist, and other interested persons hope to develop a complete leprosarium here at a cost of $150,000 to $200,000.

1955—Memorandum Radically Reshaped ALM's Program

"Our greatest desire," wrote Robert G. Cochrane, "should be the extension of the Kingdom of God, and not just doing leprosy work for the sake of charity or goodwill alone. Firstly, we must be as good as secular organizations in the technical performance of our duties, and, secondly, we must not encourage work that results in the staff being so strained that it is almost impossible either to give an effective witness or to build the Church of God.

"The three fundamental needs are in the realms of (1) Training, (2) Demonstrating, and (3) Understanding (Research). . . . so that their work shall be more effective, first, in winning souls and building up the Church, and secondly, to use their institutions in co-operative research schemes. There will always be the necessity for giving money on compassionate grounds. One must never rule out the need of the smaller institutions, however, when there is only a certain amount of money to be disposed of, priorities must be seriously considered, otherwise we will be in danger of failing in our stewardship."

1955—Dermatologist Became First Superintendent at Karigiri

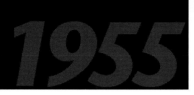

Dr. Herbert H. Gass was born in India of missionary parents. He returned to India as a qualified dermatologist and spent some years at Chandkhuri. Later, he became Professor of Dermatology at Vellore Christian Medical College, where his interest in leprosy—both as teacher and clinician—remained at the highest level. His influence on the new development at Karigiri was unmistakable. It was a natural consequence that he became the first superintendent of the William Jay Schieffelin Sanatorium, while retaining his position at Vellore and serving as the London Mission to Lepers's medical secretary for India.

1955—ALM Honored William Jay Schieffelin in Memorium

RESOLVED that this Board lay upon the record their profound appreciation of their late Chairman and President of American Leprosy Missions, Inc, William Jay Schieffelin, Ph.D., who "being dead yet liveth."

From the day in 1906, when the New York Committee of the "Mission to Lepers in India and the East" met in his home, through his election as Chairman of that Committee in 1908, and in 1920 as President of the Corporation, to his retirement as President Emeritus in 1948, Dr. Schieffelin was the unfailing friend of leprosy patients throughout the world. It was out of this simple, humane, Christian motive—personal compassion for men, women, and children who suffered—that he accepted his leadership of American Leprosy Missions. Upon it he built a structure of an exceptionally wise organization, but he never lost the warm and living consciousness of the individual.

We as Board members wish to express to that great company who by their gifts of prayer, service and money make all our work possible, and to our successors in the membership of this Board, our affectionate admiration for a leader generous in heart, spacious in mind, and irreplaceable in our history.

Dr. Schieffelin had been chairman emeritus of the Citizens Union of the City of New York and served on the board of the following organizations: American Mission to Lepers, the American Bible Society, Tuskegee Institute, and Hampton Institute. An early champion of the right of minorities, Dr. Schieffelin had a proud record of having consistently opposed oppression whether it stemmed from Munich or Mississippi.

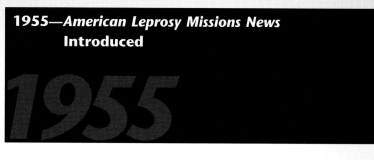

1955—American Leprosy Missions News Introduced

A new informational publication, *American Leprosy Missions News*, was introduced in 1955. A letter from the general secretary pointed out that mailed pieces such as appeal letters, news, and information would henceforth no longer originate with branch offices, but only from the New York City headquarters.

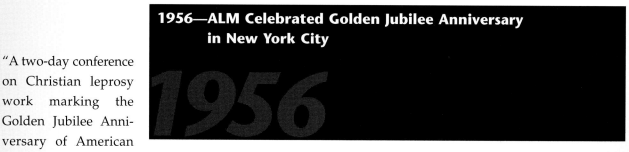

1956—ALM Celebrated Golden Jubilee Anniversary in New York City

"A two-day conference on Christian leprosy work marking the Golden Jubilee Anniversary of American Leprosy Missions will be held October 17–18, 1956, at the George Washington Hotel. Theme of the anniversary meeting will be The Role of the Christian Church in the Fight Against Hansen's Disease (Leprosy). Some 200 missionaries, doctors, and laymen interested in H.D.'s therapy are expected to attend the conference, which is one of a series to be held throughout the country during October, November and December in celebration of American Leprosy Missions' 50th birthday."

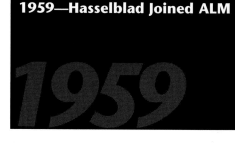

1959—Hasselblad Joined ALM

Mr. Forrest Smith, a member of the personnel committee, phoned Oliver W. Hasselblad, M.D., at Kirksville, Missouri, asking without warning: "Would you consider becoming president of American Leprosy Missions?" Dr. Hasselblad agreed to make an early visit to New York to meet the committee, resulting in his election, which took effect on June 1, 1959.

Oliver W. Hasselblad had served as a missionary physician and surgeon in India under the American Baptist Mission for almost twenty years. He was awarded the coveted Kaisar-I-Hind award from the British government for outstanding service in India. During his long service in India, Hasselblad also supervised the Kangpokpi Leprosy Hospital in Manipur for three years.

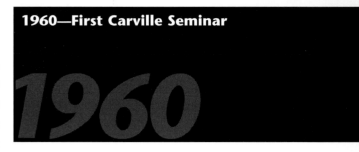

An annual seminar for leprosy workers on furlough was sponsored jointly by the United States Public Health Service (USPHS) and ALM. ALM was responsible for promoting and choosing the attendees while the Carville staff arranged the program which included overseas leprologists and lecturers. Twenty-six medical missionaries from eleven countries attended the first seminar in 1960. A year later, thirty-seven participants from more than a dozen countries attended, including a growing number of foreign medical students. Eventually, attendance was limited only by the capacity of Carville to provide accommodation. The program also included well-known Bible teachers, thus taking on the nature of a spiritual retreat. Sundays were given over to selected reports by missionaries.

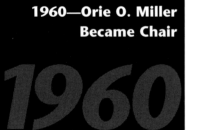

1960—Orie O. Miller Became Chair

A successful businessman, Orie O. Miller began traveling in 1919 on behalf of Mennonite and human interests. As a young man, he spent many months in relief work in Syria and Russia. A member of the board since 1958, Miller served faithfully on the ALM Executive and Overseas Committees. Long before his association with ALM, he had reflected his concern for leprosy sufferers by assisting Paraguayan Mennonites to bring Km. 81 into being with ALM help. Miller became chairman of ALM Board of Directors on October 20, 1960, and served as chairman until 1966. Writing to the ALM president in 1971, Miller stated: "I can honestly say that the past number of years connected with ALM have been the most enjoyable on my part—in fact just as enjoyable as any Mennonite Church work I have been connected with."

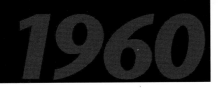

1960—Distinguished Hong Kong Researcher Visited ALM Board

Dr. Olaf K. Skinsnes of the Department of Pathology, University of Chicago (a former missionary of the Evangelical Lutheran Church in China and for some years in a research project based on the Hay Ling Chau leprosy settlement in Hong Kong), was a distinguished guest at the May 13, 1960 Board of Directors meeting. The board also considered a request for $40,711 for the University of Hawaii School of Medicine.

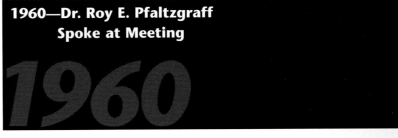

1960—Dr. Roy E. Pfaltzgraff Spoke at Meeting

At the May 13, 1960 Board of Directors meeting, Dr. Roy E. Pfaltzgraff, medical officer of the leprosy colony at Garkida, Nigeria, was a distinguished guest. The Church of the Brethren Leprosarium at Garkida unquestionably ranked as one of the best-balanced pieces of leprosy work in West Africa. Of the nearly seven thousand patients reached by its medical and spiritual ministry, more than six thousand were treated at seven outpatient clinics and segregation villages within a radius of one hundred miles. At the center of this outreach was the leprosarium, with its modern, efficient buildings, churches, and schools. An extensive evangelistic program carried the Christian message far into strongly Moslem areas. Pfaltzgraff shared this about his work:

In the spring of 1945, we went to Lassa, a station 100 miles from Garkida to do general medical work. There was a leprosy clinic there with a few patients getting hydnocarpus (chaulmoogra) oil injections. I felt that this was not very effective so I was not interested and actually never visited the clinic. However, by 1949 dapsone became available and a "segregation village" was started to care for some patients with a milder form of the disease, so that they did not need to be admitted to the "colony."

After that, I saw the efficacy of dapsone and opened another "Segregation Village" near Lassa early in 1953. Not long after, it was found reasonable to treat people in the clinics as outpatients and they no longer needed to be dislocated from their homes. New clinics were opened throughout the area and by 1962 there were 1,325 patients in outpatient care. The outpatient clinics continued to increase in numbers through the years until 1982 when we left. There were over 142 clinics in the area with over 16,000 patients on treatment.

With the transition to Government management, the name was again changed to "Gongola State Leprosy Hospital" and finally to "State Leprosy Hospital—Garkida." These name changes followed progression from custodial care to specific leprosy treatment and then to aggressive rehabilitation.

1961—Dr. Wayne Meyers Recruited

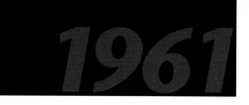

Dr. Wayne Meyers was stepping into a critical emergency caused by illness of a staff member when he was recruited to lead leprosy work at Nyankanda in Ruanda-Urundi. Unusually equipped to fill the need, Meyers had a M.D. degree from Baylor University and a Ph.D. degree in microbiology from the University of Wisconsin. He had also completed two years of training at Moody Bible Institute.

His Congo-born wife, Mrs. Esther Meyers, was a daughter of Dr. and Mrs. R. E. Kleinschmidt of the Africa Inland Mission, well known for their remarkable program in leprosy service extending from Aba in the Republic of Congo. A graduate of Wheaton College, Mrs. Meyers was familiar with African languages. Dr. and Mrs. Meyers, with their three children, left for the field immediately.

The Meyers eventually returned to the United States, where he served as pathologist at the Department of Defense. Meyers served several terms on the ALM board, including a term as chair. He also served ALM as program consultant.

1963—Wilbur Chapman Honored

On the fiftieth anniversary of the Pete the Pig Program, the board voted to establish the Wilbur Chapman Educational Fellowship Fund.

1963—Dr. Paul W. Brand Delivered Legendary Address

At the 1963 ALM Annual Meeting held at the First Baptist Church, Washington, D.C., Dr. Paul W. Brand delivered his landmark "Touch" address. Later put into pamphlet form, it had one of the widest circulations of any piece of literature produced by ALM. (see appendix D for complete text)

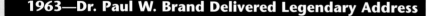

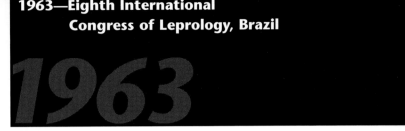

The Eighth International Congress of Leprology met in Rio de Janeiro, Brazil, with representation from more than fifty countries. A committee under the direction of missionary Dr. Hugh C. Tucker met to organize a Brazilian Mission to Lepers, representing ALM missionaries and Brazilian Protestants working in leprosaria. He served as ALM's representative until 1945, when at his suggestion the Evangelical Confederation of Brazil took over the direction of the leprosy ministry.

Over the years ALM built six chapels in government leprosaria. Several of these fine chapels were visited by Rev. Gerson A. Meyer to evaluate ALM's involvement and also to learn more about the leprosy problem in Brazil. Though ALM's interest reached far back to its early history, present marginal support appeared insufficient. The work of the chaplains, however, was excellent. Their spiritual ministry should not be minimized. With churches on the outside preparing the way, and the patients on the inside sufficiently motivated, surely many could be restored to a life of usefulness and Christian service in their own homes and communities. The possibility of a future seminar with the chaplains to set up a program of education for rehabilitation was considered, perhaps becoming one of ALM's most significant contributions.

Before such plans could be initiated, Meyer was called to Geneva to head the section of Christian education of the World Council of Churches. His greatest service to the mission was the recruitment of Rev. Jorge O. de Macedo, an ordained Baptist minister, to take up the work. CERPHA (*Comissao Evangelica de Pacientes de Hanseniase*) soon came into being, with Macedo as the executive secretary. Seed planted by the mission a great many years ago had come to fruition.

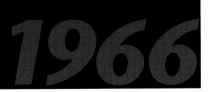

Dr. Eugene R. Kellersberger died on January 28, 1966. At the May 6, 1966, meeting of the Board of Directors, Dr. Clyde Taylor led a moving memorial tribute of Kellersberger's life and many achievements as Congo missionary and ALM general secretary for twelve years.

1966—ALM and LWM invited as Observers at European Federation of Anti-Leprosy Associations

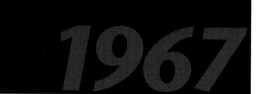

Dr. Hasselblad made supplication for admission, but membership was limited to European agencies. Soon it changed its name to ILEP, *International* Federation of Anti-Leprosy Associations, and ALM was cordially, even urgently, invited to join and has been an active member since.

1967—ALM Closed All Regional Offices

All promotion, education, and fundraising became centralized under the coordination of Osborne E. Scott, a retired military chaplain.

1967—Dr. Glen W. Tuttle Honored

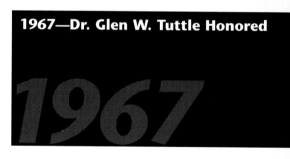

Dr. Glen W. Tuttle, retired medical missionary and "father" of the Institut Médical Evangélique (IME), at Kimpese, République Démocratique du Congo, was honored for his many years of selfless devotion and untiring efforts. He later served as ALM's administrative vice president.

1969—ALM Invited to Survey Leprosy Work in South Vietnam

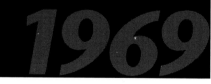

ALM received an invitation from the Vietnam Christian Service Committee to study "leprosy incidence, need and resources in South Vietnam, and make recommendations for possible U.S. church mission and service response." The program was accepted for the new unified Vietnam.

1969—Dr. Norwood B. Tye Appointed

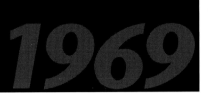

The sixty-third annual report named twenty-four persons serving overseas with full support from the mission, and announced the appointment of Norwood B. Tye as executive director of administration. Tye was a long-term missionary with the Disciples of Christ in the Philippines, where he helped bring the Philippine Leprosy Mission to maturity. Income from all sources totaled $1,385,403—the largest in ALM history.

1971—Duerksen Appointed Medical Director

Dr. Frank Duerksen was appointed medical director of Km. 81, Paraguay. The Paraguayan-born son of Mennonite immigrants from Russia, Duerksen received his medical education in Argentina and post-graduate surgical studies in Canada. Previously, he was on an ALM fellowship at ALERT studying leprosy control, rehabilitation and reparative surgery.

1972—John R. Sams Joined ALM

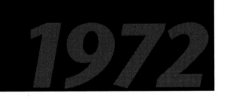

Reverend John R. Sams joined ALM as administrative vice president. A missionary in Thailand for thirteen years, and for four years in the Philippines under appointment by the Disciples of Christ, United Christian Missionary Society, much of Sams's experience had been in administrative positions. He came well qualified and had a decisive impact on the future of the mission.

1973—International Journal of Leprosy

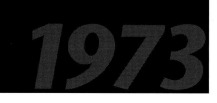

Following the Tenth International Leprosy Congress, ALM President Hasselblad reported that he had been elected executive officer of the International Leprosy Association's *International Journal of Leprosy*. Hasselblad was also elected to the council of the ILA; the undertaking was a large one, but it earned great dividends in goodwill from ILA and others.

1973—Directorship of the Schieffelin Leprosy Research & Training Center Accepted

After many hours of discussions between Dr. Ernest Fritschi, Dr. Paul Brand, and Dr. Oliver Hasselblad, agreement was reached that ALM would accept the directorship of the Schieffelin Leprosy Research & Training Center (SLR&TC) in Karigiri, India, with ALM undertaking full support for Fritschi. This arrangement assured the future of the center for a fourteen-year period extending from 1973 to 1987.

1973—Research Grant Awarded

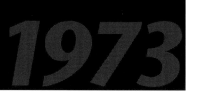

The mission was encouraged when a grant of $125,000 was received from the Victor Heiser Foundation to support three research projects:

1. The United States Public Health Service Hospital at Carville, for "exploitation of using armadillo as a laboratory animal."
2. The Department of Pathology, University of Hawaii School of Medicine, in support of research carried on by Dr. Olaf K. Skinsnes.
3. The World Health Organization for developing an International Histo-Pathology Referral Center at Caracas, Venezuela, under the direction of Dr. J. Convit.

1973—Frist Joined ALM

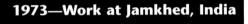

Thomas Feran Frist first came to attention when studying for a master's degree in public health at Yale University. He had requested suggestions on a field of study for his thesis, resulting in obtaining a foundation grant for the study. His well-documented thesis did, in fact, offer root causes and solutions. On the basis of it, recommendations were made to the government of Tanzania.

Frist and his wife, Clare (the daughter of Latin American missionaries), spent a year in Spain while she obtained a graduate degree in Spanish studies. An arranged period of study and observation was involved with all aspects of leprosy management in Venezuela. The Frists later performed stellar service in Brazil before Tom Frist became ALM's president, CEO in 1989.

1973—Work at Jamkhed, India

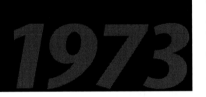

Dr. Mabelle Arole reported on the work at Jamkhed, India:

The idea of providing health care for an entire community came to us after graduation from Vellore Christian Medical College. Working in a rural health center at Vadala it was realized that curative medicine was not enough to meet the basic health needs of rural India. To this end, we came to the U.S. for further training, returning to India in 1970, each with a Masters degree in Public Health from Johns Hopkins University.

Now, in an area around Jamkhed of 54 villages with 80,000 population, a comprehensive health program provides medical services to fit the needs and economy of the community. In addition to leprosy and TB control, the rural health project includes family welfare planning and childcare, antenatal care, immunization, treatment of communicable diseases and health education.

Though a small new hospital at the Jamkhed headquarters cares for those who need temporary hospitalization, most of the work is carried on at nine health sub centers within a radius of ten miles. Mobile teams go out from Jamkhed once a month to some 15 villages in the area to serve additional multi-purpose clinics.

Village surveys and school health services are an important part of the project and have resulted in detection of early cases. In the schools, with laudable cooperation from teachers, the health team gives talks on public health, using simple, colorful posters and showing slides on leprosy. In the short time since the establishment of the health project, we have been completely accepted by the Hindu community leaders, government officials and the public, and have no problem in getting enthusiastic cooperation in the work.

1974—Inaugural Kellersberger Memorial Lecture at ALERT

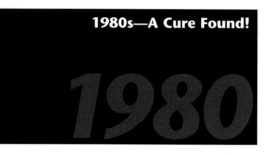

It was decided to memorialize Dr. Eugene Kellersberger in perpetuity by the establishment of an annual Kellersberger Memorial Lecture. The first lecture was given before the Ethiopian Medical Association as well as staff and trainees at ALERT by Dr. J. C. Convit, director of the International Center for Training and Research in Leprosy and Related Diseases of Caracas, Venezuela.

1980s—A Cure Found!

Scientists discovered a cocktail of three antibiotics (rifampicin, dapsone, and clofazimine) cures cases of leprosy! ALM joined an international body of leprosy organizations under direction of ILEP in distributing this powerful multidrug therapy (MDT) throughout the world.

1981-1982—MDT Became the Standard

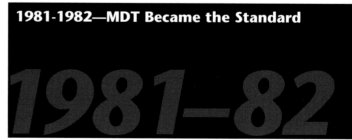

In 1981, the World Health Organization started recommending multidrug therapy, or MDT. The three drugs, taken in combination, are dapsone, rifampicin (or rifampin), and clofazimine. Treatment takes from six months to a year or more. American Leprosy Missions began using multidrug therapy in its projects in 1982. Since then, millions of people have been cured using MDT, with virtually no resistance or relapse.

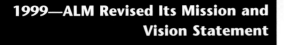

1999—ALM Revised Its Mission and Vision Statement

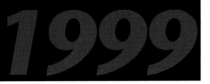

OUR MISSION
To serve as a channel of Christ's love to people with leprosy and disabilities, helping them to be healed in body and spirit and restored to lives of dignity and usefulness within their communities.

OUR VISION
Christ's servants, freeing the world of leprosy.

2003—The Search for a Vaccine Continued

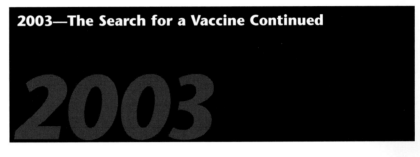

Early treatment with MDT remained the best prevention against nerve damage and deformities. There is still no vaccine against this disease, although ALM's centennial campaign seeks to fund vaccine research.

2004—Leprosy Worldwide Statistics

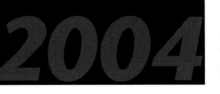

Although 14 million leprosy patients have been cured with MDT, leprosy is still present in a number of countries, especially in Africa, South Asia, and South America.

- India accounts for more than 70% of new cases.
- A further 20% of cases occur in just five countries: Brazil, Nepal, Indonesia, Bangladesh, and Myanmar (Burma).
- Seven countries in Africa account for a further 5% of new cases: Angola, D. R. Congo, Ethiopia, Madagascar, Mozambique, Nigeria, and Tanzania.

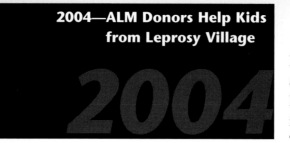

2004—ALM Donors Help Kids from Leprosy Village

In Addis Ababa, Africa, ALM donors support a tutoring project for children in one of the largest leprosy "colonies" in the world, giving about 1,200 kids hope for the future. These kids have leprosy-affected parents, and they know the experience of stigma and poverty. Many of their parents eke out their living by begging on the streets of Addis Ababa. Under the direction of Sister Senkenesh Mariam, 120 high school tutors—older children with some schooling—teach the younger children and help them to succeed. The high school tutors have gained places of honor in their villages. The pride they experience lifts them far above any dreams they could have imagined. Both the tutors and the tutored children experience the excitement that comes with education and with hope. Worldwide, ALM sponsors over one thousand children for high school, college, and technical training.

2005—ALM at Work

ALM employs approximately twenty-two people at its headquarters in Greenville, SC. This includes a doctor on staff who is the Leprosy Consultant and eight Program Overseas Personnel; approximately thirty-three people also work there as volunteers. Globally, ALM supports national programs or missions programs that are already established and trains local medical workers in the field to recognize and treat leprosy.

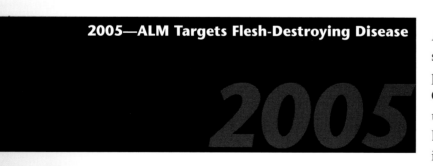

2005—ALM Targets Flesh-Destroying Disease

American Leprosy Missions has started treating Buruli ulcer patients in Ivory Coast and in Ghana. "This is a new campaign for us," said president Christopher J. Doyle. Doyle said ALM is responding to Buruli ulcer because of its aggressive and destructive nature. "In many ways it stigmatizes people as much as leprosy. It leaves them scarred and deformed. Worst of all, it affects mainly children." Buruli is a flesh-destroying bacterium that can leave large, exposed "holes" on a child's body. The only cure is expensive surgery and extended hospitalization. "This is the first time, though, our board of directors has challenged us to become intentional about finding and treating a disease other than leprosy," said Doyle. ALM will work in partnership with MAP International headquartered in Brunswick, Georgia.

ABOUT THE AUTHOR

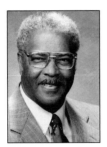 *Born in 1939, Eugene L. Wilson grew up in La Boca and Paraiso, Canal Zone, Republic of Panama. After graduating from high school, he worked as a bilingual secretary for the bishop of the Episcopal Church of the Diocese of Panama. Here, Wilson was introduced to the American Leprosy Missions through a grant for Palo Seco Leprosarium Chaplaincy.*

He married his high school sweetheart, Beverly, in 1962. The couple relocated to New York, where Eugene attended New York University. Wilson's application for employment with the Episcopal Church was referred to American Leprosy Missions. Thus began a thirty-nine-year career that included service as ALM's office manager, controller, and director of program finance and administration, before ending with retirement in 2001. He also represented ALM on the Board of the American Council on Gift Annuities for more than twenty-five years.

While living in Cambria Heights, New York, he was active in a variety of community, civic, political, and church organizations. As president of a community association, he helped supervise sports activities for youth and initiated an after-school tutorial program through grants from the city and state of New York. The organization was recognized in a legislative proclamation in the New York State Assembly. Wilson also chaired the Finance Committee of Cambria Heights St. David's Episcopal Church.

Wilson and his wife, Beverly, now reside in Florida. Their two grown children and three grandchildren live in Texas and New York.

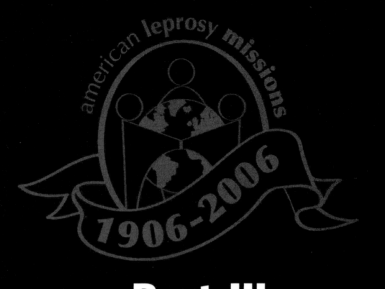

Part III

Chapter 7

Stigma Destroys the Spirit

by Hugh Cross

When the women of the village in Mahottari gather at the well, they appear from a distance like a flock of exotic birds. The bright sarees flutter as their arms dip and hoist to pull buckets from the well. They chatter, nudge each other, and laugh. It is a little lighthearted relief from the drudge and monotony of life in a Maithili village.

When outsiders approach the group, Lagaan Devi lurks behind the mango tree. She doesn't jostle with the rest. She doesn't nudge and joke about her friends' cooking. She waits until the others have finished, then she draws water, alone. As the other women shuffle off to their houses, their feet patter as sandals slap their heels. Lagaan Devi wears ugly green canvas shoes, a sure giveaway that she has foot ulcers. Everybody in the village knows that she has leprosy. They distrust her. The local term for one with leprosy in her village is *khoeri*, which means curse. Her presence, it is feared, will be a misfortune to others.

When Lagaan Devi had been hospitalized for treatment, we discovered that she was being treated savagely. Her face veiled behind a fold of her saree, she told us in broken whispers how the villagers beat her and threw stones at her. They did not allow her to draw water from the well and she was forbidden to walk on the road. Eventually Lagaan Devi was discharged from the hospital and with great trepidation she returned to her village, but on this occasion, we accompanied her.

When we arrived, we explained leprosy to the village leaders and asked for their help in restoring Lagaan Devi to her role in the village. We deliberately attracted attention to ourselves so the neighbors would see us taking food and tea from her hand. We listened to their fears and talked about her everyday reality. We left feeling confident that the village accepted our arguments and that they were willing to accept Lagaan Devi back into village life.

Not many months later she returned to the hospital for treatment of a different problem. Her bearing was more erect. She wore bangles. Her gestures were lively. She scolded her small child with all the pride of any Maithili mother who has a son to display. She greeted us with warm familiarity and after the expected preamble we asked if life had changed for her since we met in her village. "Oh yes!" she said without hesitation, "it is now much better, the men don't beat me any more, now they only spit at me." I guess distress is relative.

The word leprosy, when spoken, can have an effect as strong as the sight of deformity. Most people who suffer leprosy never develop deformities, and most are indistinguishable from the people we pass in the street. Nonetheless, an individual who suffers from "leprosy" experiences the discrimination reserved for those who offend society.

Stigma

Through the millennia, since Jesus' ascension, there have been reports that certain people:

saints and hermits, shepherds and schoolgirls, have exhibited wounds that appeared spontaneously, without explanation. The wounds characteristically appear on the same sites on the body that Jesus' wounds were known to have been. These miraculous presentations (genuine or bogus) were termed "stigmata," roughly translated "the marks." The stigmata were the label that signified that the person who bore them was "different"; they were distinctive and usually assumed to have miraculous or paranormal powers. Saint Francis of Assisi is perhaps one famous person who apparently exhibited stigmata. How is it, then, that when plural, "stigmata" has a positive meaning, but the singular "stigma" is so negative?

Stigma is a many-barbed phenomenon. It can come from a society trying to protect itself. It can even start as a voluntary action by an affected individual who decides he should withdraw because he has become different. He fears he could threaten the stability of family and community. Stigma nearly always provokes rejection and hostility, but it is just as likely to stimulate compassion. Leprosy workers work hard to erase the negative affects of stigma, but when we truly examine our practices, the dreadful reality is that very often we perpetuate it. Stigma experts use different terms to identify types of stigma and the different effects of the phenomenon.

Enacted Stigma

"Enacted stigma" describes situations where someone with leprosy is actively discriminated against, as illustrated by Lagaan Devi. Why did the men in Lagaan Devi's village continue to spit at her? Probably because she was considered cursed. The people could understand that germs caused the disease and that it could be treated. They probably even accepted that she would not infect others. What we could not explain to their satisfaction is why she was the one to get the disease in the first place. Why her and not one of the other women who chatter at the well?

Perceived Stigma

"Enacted stigma" is straightforward: People are afraid of someone with leprosy so they exclude them to protect themselves. "Perceived stigma," however, is perhaps more difficult to detect and almost certainly more difficult to overcome.

All cultures, according to sociologists, have belief systems that explain the mysteries of life. They are not taught formally. They are learned from our parents and peers in the process of growing up.

Children grow up observing that leprosy is dreaded and that there are legitimate actions to be taken against those who have it. In some cultures, hostile actions are thought to be deserved because leprosy and the hostility it evokes is considered just punishment for wrongdoing either in this life or a previous life. Other cultures hold that someone's affliction is due to unwholesome or antisocial behavior. Others consider leprosy to be a consequence of class that suggests inferior breeding. In cultures with a strong sense of guilt and punishment, such beliefs create a desperate dilemma for one who suddenly develops the disease. A diagnosis of leprosy is a serious challenge to someone's self image. The negative psychological impact can far outweigh the physical effects of the disease.

Myanmar has a highly effective health delivery system, the backbone of which is midwives. With bright white blouses and scarlet skirts they bounce over the rough roads of rural Myanmar on red bicycles. Affectionately known as the "Red Angels," they proudly take health delivery literally to the doors of the sick. Amongst other duties, they are entrusted with health education and community awareness programs. I have had many opportunities to engage the Red Angels and supporting NGOs in discussions about leprosy. Not only are they determined, their attitudes always seem positive.

The Red Angels report that in their communities, the attitude towards those who had leprosy were generally positive. Myanmar is one country where the problem of enacted stigma does not appear to exist. One might hope that in such a climate of acceptance, people with leprosy might cope with the disease far more positively. Perceived stigma, however, seems to confound that hope.

I have been in conversations with people in other parts of Myanmar where I was told that persons with leprosy had been treated poorly. They left their homes and families not wanting to bring hardship on them.

One young man is particularly memorable. I met him at a rural health center he had been compelled to attend because a program evaluation team was scheduled to visit. He was in a sad state of self-neglect. He was filthy; ulcers consumed his young feet. I noticed his fixed attention on a spot on the floor. He flicked irritably at his knee. The vacancy and monotony of his actions told us quite plainly that he would rather not speak to us. We carefully navigated a conversation, taking care not to touch on sensitive subjects.

We learned that he had left his father's home voluntarily and chose to stay with an uncle who gave him food in exchange for work. He was a threat and a burden, repulsive to others and to himself, trapped in a destructive spiral that led to self-neglect and physical deterioration. His uncontrolled physical deterioration and self-loathing eroded any reason to look after himself. If he looked to the future, he could only see loneliness and destitution. Without realizing what he was doing, he had adopted the identity of a leper and was rapidly transforming himself to fit the role.

Self Stigma

"Self stigma" is another form of perceived stigma. When individuals lose control over their decisions and actions, they are in danger of losing self-esteem. As they lose self-esteem they begin to fall into cycles of depression, believing that they are hopeless and unworthy. They withdraw from social contact. Not because they feel that they may be a threat; rather, they lose confidence that they have any right to be included in the schemes and activities of others. This is one reason why it is so

important for health workers to include people affected by leprosy in every aspect of their treatment. The problem of exclusion leading to low self-esteem is more acute in authoritarian cultures.

Hindu cultures have a very strong element of ritual with very clearly drawn roles within the family structure. There is no traditional role for an individual in isolation. Everybody fits into a structure that strives for the benefit of the family as a unit. With its strong emphasis on purity and ritual, a case of leprosy can cause a huge family dilemma.

In a strong concept of family, decisions are often made for individual members, particularly women. A decision by family leaders to adopt isolation is accepted by the victim. For example, a beautiful, well-educated young woman has three very caring elder brothers. A chartered architect, she has the poise and grace of a model, but without arrogance. It is difficult to detect that she had leprosy, except that on very close examination it could be seen that the small muscles that control her left thumb had partially wasted. Any prospective mother-in-law would surely notice this imperfection. The girl would subsequently be rejected as a potential bride, and the family would be humiliated. The brothers eventually accept that nothing could be done to restore the atrophied muscle to a more plump appearance and make the tragic decision not to seek a husband for their sister.

Many researchers have studied stigma to determine the main actors in leprosy drama. The affected person is obviously the principal player. The late Professor Valencia was an eminent Filipino academic who had an interest in this problem. She suggested that stigma is as much a disease as leprosy. Leprosy may damage the body, but stigma damages character. She went so far as to say: "The disease is perceived as one that uglifies not only the body but the soul; it turns, though slowly, a person into a thing." The dehumanizing effects of the disease can make the person fearful to others and loathsome to himself.

Dr. E. Gofman presented a lot of groundbreaking work on the subject of stigma. Since his time, many sociologists and anthropologists have studied different aspects of the issue. Most sociologists agree that people "learn to become lepers," so who are the teachers? One of the most startling conclusions is that stigma is partly the result of actions from a group that might be least expected—health workers!

In many countries, the care of people with leprosy was traditionally a ministry for nuns. These dedicated sisters ministered to the needs of those with leprosy with tireless devotion. Tireless devotion would seem to be an admirable quality, but not, as some sociologists have explained, if it leads to people eventually believing they can do nothing for themselves. The care that the nuns gave was so complete that those who had leprosy would, in time, yield almost every function to the care of the nuns.

Through their actions, though well intended, the nuns taught the people they ministered to that they were different, that they needed to be cared for, that they needed the love of the nuns because they were rejected by others. The loving attention created a complete dependency on the nuns to the extent that the leprosy-affected people believed they were

The Jamkhed Project

Gangubai's mother-in-law confiscated her leprosy medicine. Then she confined her daughter-in-law to a corner room. For a year, the young woman stayed trapped and alone while the family hoped she would die. Her husband abandoned her completely. The only visitors she had were her two young daughters. Only they wanted their mother cured. They convinced their mother she must live.

Gangubai set up a secret meeting with the village health worker (VHW) whom her mother-in-law had forbidden in her house. The VHW took Gangubai to the Jamkhed leprosy center (funded with ALM gifts), and that's where she began her new life.

At Jamkhed, Gangubai was treated for her leprosy. She also received three small loans, fifteen goats, some poultry, a sewing machine, and tailoring lessons. She even received daily bus money to attend training classes.

Soon, she was raising and selling more goats and poultry. She sold colorful bangles, as well. She repaid all three loans.

"Without the village health worker, I would have died long ago," she says. "Leprosy deformities would have forced me out of my village and onto the streets. I would have spent my last days begging and then dying unnoticed."

Today Gangubai is a new creation with a renewed faith in God. She says, "The Jamkhed Project is one of His blessings. It brought me out of misery and illness and into a new and better life."

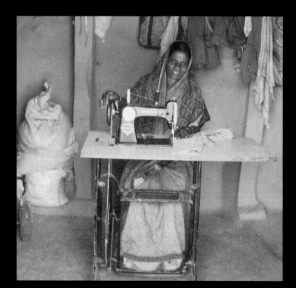

useless and worthless, except as objects for others to practice their charity.

An essential part of human dignity is being allowed to contribute. The sisters were able to enjoy this privilege abundantly while the people they ministered to dwindled into complete dependency and lack of self-esteem. Those who studied the situation have pointed out that the nuns actually needed the people affected by leprosy just as much as the people who were dependent on them. Working with lepers gave them a raison d'être. Some researchers have called this effect "leprophilia" which means a love of leprosy.

The sad truth is that exactly the same effect can still be seen throughout the world in well-intentioned evangelical missions. Most who have worked in leprosy hospitals or similar institutions know the desperate appeal not to be discharged because someone has come to depend on the loving attention given to them in the confines of a hospital.

I had to learn this lesson myself. Compassion must on occasions also be tough. Compassion seeks the best for others rather than satisfying one's own emotions. It is very rewarding to sit at the feet of somebody who has suffered. The reality, though, is that such people need to be equipped to face the hard knocks of life where they won't have the luxury of daily ministrations and emotional support. They need to be able to walk into their villages, fully convinced that they are not hopeless, dependent lepers. Even leprous beggars can change their appearance and make a useful contribution.

Exploited Stigma

Some who show the signs of leprosy have strong reasons for maintaining a negative self-image. They are beggars who depend on their disfigurement and disability for alms.

There seems to be a threshold of dignity that prevents people from succumbing to the image of the "leprosy beggar." There comes a point when people deformed by leprosy become almost hard-ened to negative attitudes and exclusion. When this point is reached, there can be a turning from rejecting their label to exploiting it. It is not an easy transition. I have interviewed professional beggars who felt ashamed to admit their role.

Kushi Das died a few years ago. To most who saw him, he was just another beggar at the side of the road. Ironically, he probably made more contact with others than do the vast majority of Nepalese people. Passersby in Kathmandu, or Janakpur, Delhi, Allahabad, or Patna, were moved by his begging pitch, and tossed him a few coins. He was better traveled than most Nepalese people. Kushi was fleetingly seen and instantly forgotten. He taught me as much about leprosy as did some persons I had worked with for many years. He was like so many thousands who understand the cruelty of exclusion, but his eloquence and honesty made conversation particularly revealing.

From time to time Kushi had resorted to begging and joined the many thousands that cluster around temples and mosques throughout South Asia. He had learned to put a value on his deformities and knew how to display them to best advantage. In quiet interviews, away from other ears, he told my colleague and me how the beggars of Kathmandu were organized. People with the shared identity of leprosy who have been rejected from their communities not uncommonly seek the companionship of each other. Even though they are generally considered to be deviants, the groups of beggars that I have known have developed their own societies with their own rules and regulations, sometimes more rigorously upheld and administered than those in wider society.

In illustrating this, Kushi giggled nervously and confided in a sort of raucous whisper how beggars meet at night to discuss the best locations to display different deformities and disabilities. The blind drew sympathy in some locations while those with ulcers did not. Deformed hands were always useful. Babies, of course, drew coins out of pockets anywhere, but it helped if a woman with deformed hands carried the baby.

This sometimes meant lending a baby to those who could use them to best effect.

Ulcers always caused distress and if somebody who showed alarm could be pursued they would often pay just to be left alone. Dirty bandages would be kept and their potency would be enhanced by a splash of sugar water to attract the flies. Before leaving for work in the mornings the theatrical bandages would be wrapped around hands and feet that often never had ulcers at all. Kushi told us unashamedly that they would sit together at night and laugh about the idiots who had been fooled into emptying their pockets. Though he never said it, he believed that since they were stigmatized anyway, they might as well exploit it.

Altering Attitudes

Creating a strong self-image is only one part of the battle against stigma. There is still the huge problem of how the general public

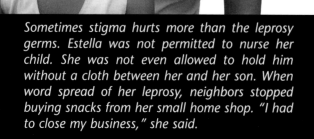

Sometimes stigma hurts more than the leprosy germs. Estella was not permitted to nurse her child. She was not even allowed to hold him without a cloth between her and her son. When word spread of her leprosy, neighbors stopped buying snacks from her small home shop. "I had to close my business," she said.

perceives leprosy and those who suffer because of it. If stigma were a straightforward problem of ignorance, then it would be logical to assume that sound arguments and well-presented information would dispel fears. Tackling the problem, however, is fraught with difficulty, partly because the stigma of leprosy is not wholly rational.

In 1998 the Nepal Leprosy Trust conducted a survey of attitudes, knowledge, and practice in an area of Nepal known to carry a heavy burden of leprosy. After the first survey was completed, the Trust carried out an intensive community awareness program. Teams of well-trained street performers went from village to village to perform plays. The simple message was that leprosy is only mildly contagious, that treatment is free and easily available, and that once started on treatment, people who have the disease do not infect others. The lively plays were acted out on dusty roads amongst the clamor of bicycles, buffaloes, and buses. They drew large attentive crowds. It was entertainment laced with easily digested information which not only increased knowledge, but also resulted in less hostile attitudes toward those who suffer it.

On completion of the awareness program, a second survey found that people really did have a much better knowledge of the disease and its treatment. It was also learned, however, that knowledge was not the great liberator everyone had hoped. Sadly, it was found that people still did not allow their children to sit near anybody with signs of leprosy. Nor would they eat with someone who had the disease. And they certainly wouldn't let their children marry into a family with a history of leprosy.

Perhaps an even more shocking example of how irrational stigma is can be found in the Philippines where leprosy was a significant problem after the Second World War. A concerted effort was undertaken to get the problem under control. No effective treatment was available at the time, but it was thought that the most effective method of controlling the disease was to incarcerate affected people in remote sanatoria.

Princess Diana and TLMI

In 1991, Her Royal Highness The Princess of Wales (Diana) attended a World Leprosy Day Service in Peterborough Cathedral, marking her first official appearance as Patron of The Leprosy Mission International of Great Britain.

Over the next several years, she was to visit TLMI projects around the world. Following her visit to a hospital in Nepal, a doctor commented, "The Princess's visit has proved that people don't have to be worried or scared about leprosy—that you can sit down and touch patients as the Princess did."

Her personal and loving touch remains one of the Princess's special legacies. She focused the world's attention on this tragic disease; and she treated each person she met—even Karna, a maimed beggar—with affection and dignity.

—**Susan S. Renault**

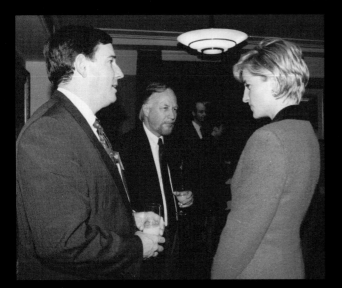

The late Princess Diana was a good friend to those with leprosy. Here, she greets ALM President Christopher Doyle while Bert Zeilhaus looks on.

With our privileged perspective of hindsight, it is easy to criticize the actions taken, but in accordance with the wisdom of that time, there was no other choice. It was a desperate measure to control a desperate problem. Eight sanatoria were established and many thousands lived out their lives in them. The sanatoria still exist today, but now that leprosy is no longer considered to be a significant public health problem, the sanatoria have extended their services to the general population.

It was hoped that by opening the sanatoria services to the general public, stigma would be dispelled. The integration of services has certainly helped, but it was at one of the sanatoria that I encountered an exasperating example of stigma. The hospital at the sanitarium in question had accepted general patients who were occupying many of the bed spaces. The hospital was, however, still mandated to serve the requirements of people affected by leprosy.

Among the people who came for admission were elderly people who once had leprosy and continued to have some telltale deformities of the disease. The tragedy I encountered was a policy of segregating a person who once had leprosy (decades ago) and later developed one of the more common ailments associated with old age. Not only were they required to stay in a separate ward, but they were also allocated their own staff because general nurses were unwilling to treat them. They had become isolated in the very place that had been set aside for them.

If it isn't knowledge—or the lack of it—that erodes or maintains stigma, then what is the problem? There are anthropologists who are working on this problem and, it is hoped, when we know the full answer, we can begin to tackle its source. As I have spoken to people and have asked them what it is about leprosy that they dislike, the answers usually revolve around the same theme. People are repulsed by ulceration and deformity. They don't fear the disease per se. They fear the visible effects of the disease.

People find it hard to trust others who are different or who belong to another group. Humans need to feel secure; anything that rocks the boat is threatening. It is a primeval defense mechanism that continues to affect human judgment. If people look different, they appear to be threatening. When threatened, we respond by showing hostility. In the case of people deformed by leprosy (stigmatized), hostility is manifested as rejection. Just as it makes no sense to consider a person with a different skin color as a threat, so it also makes no sense to consider a person of a different shape as a threat. The most difficult fear to combat, it seems, is a fear that is not rational.

So the question remains: How can we respond to the challenge stigma presents? Stigma is dehumanizing; it suggests that people do not belong. Perhaps the answer lies with people affected by leprosy themselves.

Stigma Elimination Program

An innovative program is currently underway in Nepal. Stigma Elimination Program (STEP) is a project under the supervision of the Nepal Leprosy Trust. The Trust decided to try a new approach to community development. The idea is that people affected by leprosy will be trained as change agents in their villages. Ten people were recognized as having leadership potential, though some were illiterate. All had experienced the effects of stigma.

I was particularly encouraged by one group I found on a recent visit to Nepal. Starting as a group of eight, they had grown to twenty-five. Through the literacy program they initiated, many were able to read and write with enough skill to negotiate bank loans and trade effectively. As the literacy classes grew in size and reputation, many village children tried to sneak in to take advantage of the classes. They were denied regular education either because their parents were poor or because they belonged to the untouchable caste. Understanding the plight of these children, the group negotiated with their teacher to give the children their own class. At the time of my visit twenty children were enrolled and at least another twenty were waiting to join.

The village leaders have recognized the positive affects the group is having on village life and have requested that the group leader attend all village development meetings. His advice is sought and his voice is heard and respected. In his own words, the group leader explained to me that, "the leprosy stigma has not yet disappeared but it is about seventy-five percent gone." A year ago that man was suffering humiliation and rejection. He could imagine nothing to hope for other than to be left alone. Now he is an active participant in the affairs of the village and, thanks to him, a group of children who would never have had the opportunity to learn to read are reciting their lessons and writing letters on slates.

When people affected by leprosy are given an opportunity to demonstrate their humanity (rather than seek to benefit from the humanity of others), the communities in which they live—and the world in general—will celebrate their diverse abilities. Then, and only then will we be able to say that leprosy has been eradicated.

ABOUT THE AUTHOR

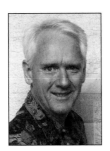

*D*r. Hugh Cross has served as ALM's regional Prevention of Disability (POD) Asia coordinator since 2003. An early achievement was to design a diploma course featuring podiatric therapies for leprosy, diabetes, and rheumatoid arthritis.

Cross has published articles in Leprosy Review and contributed a chapter to Disorders of the Foot *published by Churchill Livingstone. In 2003, he published* Wound Care For People Affected by Leprosy: A Guide for Low Resource Situations, *published in the Philippines by ALM. This guide deals with the normal body response to tissue damage and advocates the use of simple treatment methods to assist the body to repairing itself.*

Cross was born and lived in Zimbabwe, then Rhodesia. He moved to the United Kingdom in 1975, and worked as a shepherd for fifteen years in Scotland and Northern England. At age thirty-nine, he went to Queen Margaret College in Edinburgh and graduated with distinction, earning a degree in podiatry followed by a Ph.D. After a year of consultancy work for Nepal Leprosy Trust, the Leprosy Mission, and other leprosy organizations, Cross spent four years directing programs at Lalgadh Leprosy Services Centre in the Nepal Terai. Hugh Cross and his wife, Diana, reside in the Philippines. Their three adult sons live in the United Kingdom.

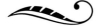

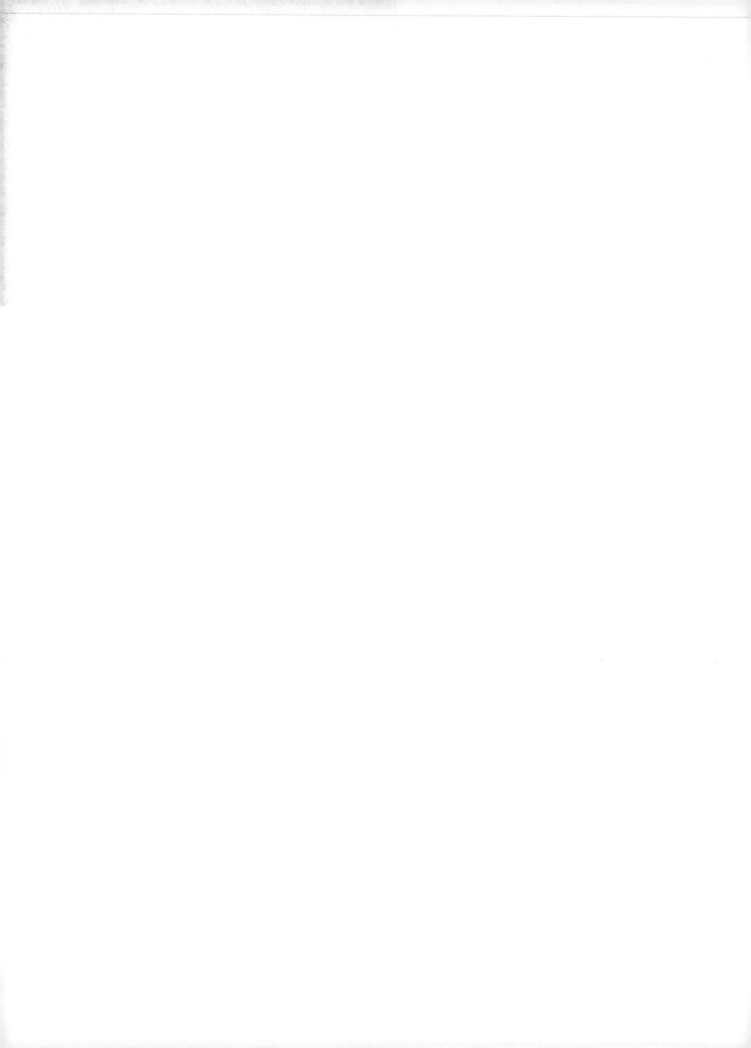

Chapter 8

Research: From Divine Curse to Scientific Conundrum

by David Scollard

Leprosy has proven to be an extraordinary puzzle for medical research. The list of doctors and scientists who have attempted to solve this puzzle includes some of the most respected names in medical research, some working on it throughout their careers. Many, however became frustrated and redirected their attention to subjects where success was more quickly achievable.

Much progress has been made. Treatments are at long last available to cure the infection and repair many of the deformities and disabilities. Yet some basic questions remain unsolved, such as how the disease is transmitted and how it can be prevented. How is the causative factor expressed or, in modern scientific terms, what mechanisms are involved? Some of these questions have been answered, while others remain a mystery.

The medical understanding of leprosy began in Norway, where leprosy was prevalent in the 1800s. Two Norwegian doctors, Daniel Cornelius Danielssen and Carl Wilhelm Boeck, published an illustrated *Atlas of Leprosy* in 1847. In it they demonstrated for the first time that patients with many different appearances had the same disease, thus beginning the scientific process of recognizing leprosy.

Their achievement provided the first explanation for the cause of leprosy and is essential in research and treatment today. Because members of the same family were often afflicted, it was widely—though mistakenly—believed to be hereditary. Soon a new explanation was provided, but the idea of "something hereditary" percolates through research up to the present day, in a more subtle and complex manner.

The second major advance in leprosy research also originated in Norway when Gerhard Armauer Hansen was the medical officer for a large leprosarium near Bergen, then Norway's largest city. Hansen was inspired by the new germ theory of disease. These tiny organisms were observed through primitive microscopes, but only anthrax was thought to be caused by a germ. Anthrax is an animal disease which occasionally affects workers who handle cattle or hides. The prevailing medical and scientific opinion was that humans and animals were biologically different and therefore germs seldom caused important human diseases. Anthrax was thought to be an exception.

Undeterred, Hansen examined biopsies from the skin of leprosy patients. He astounded the medical societies of Europe when, in 1874, he reported finding small, rod-shaped bacilli in biopsies that he proposed were germs causing leprosy. His proposal was met with great skepticism, notably by Professor Danielssen, his father-in-law.

The *Atlas of Leprosy*, 1847

Norwegian doctors Danielssen and Boeck were the first to recognize that patients with very different appearances actually had the same disease—leprosy. They described patients as having the "nodular" or the "neural" type of leprosy. This marks the first important step in understandings that would eventually lead to the modern classification of leprosy.

The idea gained acceptance when Hansen later conferred with a young German scientist, Albert Neisser, a student of Dr. Robert Koch who had described the bacilli causing tuberculosis. Neisser and others confirmed Hansen's original observations. There was a temporary controversy over who should get the credit, but the organism was eventually given the scientific name *Mycobacterium leprae* (*M. leprae*), but even today it is commonly referred to as Hansen's disease.

This landmark achievement contributed to the birth of modern medical microbiology. Many advances in understanding, preventing, and treating other infectious diseases have resulted from the ability to culture the causative organisms and grow them in the artificial media of a laboratory. *M. leprae* resisted Hansen's original efforts to cultivate it, however, and this difficulty has dogged leprosy research since.

From the time of Hansen's discovery until the mid–1960s, leprosy research was concentrated in four major areas: the causative organism, *M. leprae*; a common basis on which to classify the many diverse features of this disease; detailed descriptions of the lesions in the skin and other organs; and finding a cure for leprosy.

Soon after Hansen's discovery, controversy arose over the means of transmission, hindered by the inability to culture it in the laboratory. These gaps in medical knowledge heightened fear of leprosy, then believed to be a highly contagious disease. The ancient fear of leprosy as a curse was replaced by an inordinate fear of contagion.

A German-Brazilian scientist, Alfredo Lutz, believed strongly that transmission was by mosquitoes, following the precedent of malaria and yellow fever. Dr. Robert Cochrane disproved this theory with the finding that in India persons in adjacent villages but of different castes (and therefore having no direct physical contact), had very different rates of leprosy, while the rates for malaria were the same in all groups, regardless of caste.

Others looked to tuberculosis for a precedent. Some germs could be carried on clothing or personal items ("fomites," in medical terminology) while others became infected by contact, leading some to suspect that this might also be true of *M. leprae*.

Popular scientific understanding (or *misunderstanding*) may have unpredictable and tragic consequences. In this case, the fear of contagion led to fumigating or burning the clothing or houses of persons infected by leprosy. Letters were disinfected. Patients were physically separated from visiting family members by barriers or glass partitions to prevent touching. Newborn babies were separated from their mothers. Some countries printed special currency for use only within leprosy colonies. Early studies and speculations generated much heated debate but little light.

In the midst of such fears and frustrations, the scientific spotlight shifted to the central Philippines. Dr. James Doull, renowned for his studies of the transmission of tuberculosis, teamed up with Filipino colleagues, particularly Dr. Ricardo Guinto, in the 1930s. Employing the discipline of epidemiology, with a staff of nurses and field workers they meticulously documented the prevalence of leprosy in small towns and fishing villages where life was relatively stable.

When they returned to a village where previously no cases of leprosy had been found, they discovered one fisherman with leprosy. Subsequently they learned that he had recently moved into the village. No curative treatment was available, and fear of being sent to a leprosarium commonly caused patients to flee. They decided to provide care for patients within their own village, and in the process they could follow all of the residents carefully. Caretakers, too, were susceptible and without cure.

This is probably the best study ever done to describe the epidemiology of leprosy. They

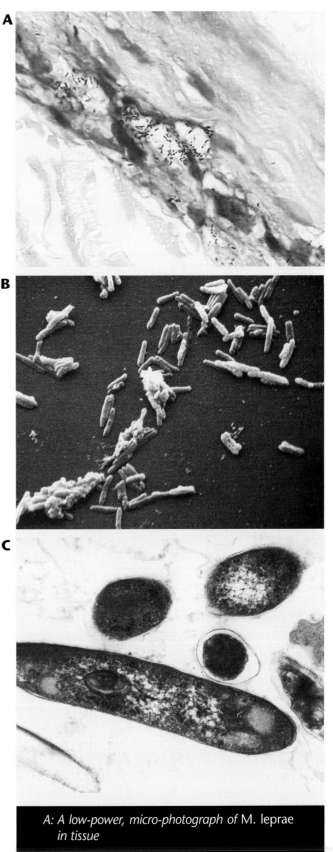

A: A low-power, micro-photograph of M. leprae in tissue

B: A high-power, micro-photograph of M. leprae

C: An electron microscope photo of M. leprae

collected and recorded their information so carefully that nearly seventy years later another epidemiologist, Dr. Paul Fine, was able to reexamine their data and look for new clues with statistical methods not available to the original investigators.

Doull and Guinto found that leprosy was more common in men than in women; that children were more susceptible than adults. But most important, they observed that leprosy spread more slowly than tuberculosis or most other diseases. Prolonged, close contact with a patient was a major risk factor in transmission, and the risk was much greater if contact was with a patient who had a large number of skin bacilli. Their work had thus demonstrated that, although leprosy is an infectious disease, it is not as contagious as generally believed. Some truths are accepted very slowly, however, and even today it is necessary to stress that it is relatively difficult to contract leprosy. The careful observations of Doull and Guinto, however, still were unable to determine how leprosy was transmitted.

For nearly a century after Hansen's discovery, in the face of continuing inability to cultivate *M. leprae* in the laboratory, research concentrated primarily on detailed studies of clinical and pathologic types of lesions and on determining which organs were or were not involved. From the late 1800s to the mid-1900s, some giants of the developing medical specialty of pathology applied their considerable skills toward an understanding of leprosy: Virchow in Germany, Mitsuda in Japan, Khanolkar in India, and many others.

In addition to the obvious involvement of the skin, peripheral nerves were quickly identified as major sites of infection. It became increasingly apparent that this was a unique property of this bacillus. Although some viruses selectively involve nerves, no other bacteria are able to do so. Why and how *M. leprae* infects nerves remains a subject of scientific inquiry. These observations regarding infection of nerves nevertheless provided valuable information and began to explain the clinical findings of nerve-related injury—loss of sensation, muscle weakness, and ultimately anesthesia, paralysis, and deformity.

Similarly, pathologists peering into their microscopes discovered that the major cell within which leprosy bacilli appeared to thrive and proliferate is, in fact, the cell that should have been its most potent killer. This cell is called the *macrophage,* and because *M. leprae* is so well adapted to live within it, it is regarded as one of a small number of intracellular parasites.

Starting in 1897, leprosy scientists and doctors have met every five years. Although the painstaking effort to grow *M. leprae* in the lab has been a topic of debate, until the 1950s concentration was on combining clinical and pathological findings into a classification system. Such a system would enable physicians to determine which patients truly have leprosy and what the prognosis is for patients whose symptoms and medical findings conform to a particular grouping.

The many different clinical manifestations of leprosy and a similar variety of appearances under the microscope puzzled and frustrated attempts to find an all-inclusive system of classification. Additionally, it was soon evident that the combinations of clinical and pathological types of leprosy varied between races and continents. This made it difficult for researchers working in Africa to accurately compare their findings with those in Asia, Europe, or South America. It was clear that leprosy was caused by *M. leprae,* but a *common thread* tying together all the disparate manifestations of the disease was elusive. Leprosy remained an enigma.

The next major step was not so much a laboratory discovery as the successful intellectual synthesis of the microbiology and pathology of leprosy, and the newly emerging discipline of immunology—the study of how the body defends itself. Earliest research in immunology focused on antibodies, proteins that circulate in the bloodstream and provide a significant mechanism of defense against many infectious agents that cause disease (pathogens).

All effective vaccines available today provide protection by stimulating the body to produce specific antibodies that enable rapid inactivation and killing of a bacterial or viral pathogen. A few major pathogens are not hindered by antibodies, however—*M. tuberculosis* and *M. leprae* are among them. Research on tuberculosis during the middle of the last century demonstrated that effective defense against this pathogen depended on the direct action of defensive cells, white blood cells. Such immunity was called "cell-mediated" or "cellular immunity."

Combining the available knowledge of cellular immunity with the pathology and microbiology of leprosy, Dr. Olaf Skinsnes, an American, wrote a landmark chapter entitled "The Immunological Spectrum of Leprosy" in Cochrane and Davey's 1964 classic text, *Leprosy in Theory and Practice*. Here Skinsnes put forward the theoretical framework that had eluded scientists for nearly a century—*the common thread being the immune response*.

Leprosy is *caused* by *M. leprae*, but the diverse appearances in different patients are the result of *differing immunity* between them. Persons with strong cellular immunity have, as a result, very few bacilli in their bodies, and have the clinical lesions that Danielssen and Boeck had described as "neural." Because of its microscopic similarities to lesions in tuberculosis, this was called "tuberculoid."

Patients with almost no immunity to the leprosy bacillus have, as a result, enormous numbers of bacilli, and they develop what Danielssen and Boeck called "nodular," now renamed "lepromatous." Moreover, all the other types of leprosy can be found in between these two extremes, forming a continuous series or spectrum of immunity. This sorting out process also revealed to immunologists everywhere that leprosy represented the most remarkable example of such an immunologic spectrum in human medicine.

Soon after Cochrane and Davey's text was published, two doctors in England, Denis Ridley and W. H. Jopling, provided a practical five-part classification system based upon the same concept that enabled physicians and pathologists from anywhere in the world to classify leprosy according to the same criteria. This permitted them to accurately compare information. Today, all studies concerning treatment, immunity, genetics, and candidate vaccines in human leprosy use this classification system as the yardstick by which to determine if the new information fits what is known about the clinical disease. Research has also shown that all new drugs (and new combinations of drugs) for leprosy are best prescribed in accordance with this spectrum—patients with less immunity need more medicine and for a longer time.

Leprosy is found worldwide, thus research into its many facets is correspondingly global. Ancient Burmese legends held that the oil of the chaulmoogra tree was beneficial in treating leprosy. In the early 1900s, this traditional remedy was rediscovered by British physicians in India. The American physician, Dr. Victor Heiser, later popularized it.

Was This the Long-Awaited Cure?

Cuttings of chaulmoogra trees soon appeared in leprosy hospitals and botanical gardens everywhere. Clinical studies attempted to determine if the oil was more effective if taken orally or by injection. Injections of chaulmoogra oil appeared for a time to be beneficial, and the major pharmaceutical company, Eli Lilly, produced and marketed it.

Leprosy hospitals were finally able to discharge patients from what had been lifetime quarantine. The injections were very painful, however—elderly patients who received them in their youth still recall them vividly and describe the experience in animated terms. Chaulmoogra oil did not, to the grave disappointment of many, provide any benefit for most patients, and for those who appeared to be helped, it was temporary.

Try, Try Again!

Then in the early 1940s, half way around the world from the chaulmoogra forests of Burma, the most far-reaching developments in the history of leprosy emerged from a hospital nestled in a wide bend of the Mississippi River. The United States Marine Hospital No. #66, later known as the U.S. Public Health Service Hospital near Carville, Louisiana.

It was here that Dr. Guy Faget and his colleagues pursued the testing of drugs intended for the treatment of tuberculosis. Since *M. tuberculosis* was readily cultivated in the laboratory, large numbers of candidate drugs could be tested. Drugs that showed promise could be prepared and tested, permitting scientists to methodically identify those most toxic to the germ and least toxic to laboratory animals. Faget tried promin, a sulfone drug that had been developed in this way but not found to be highly effective against tuberculosis.

While the world was consumed by World War II, Carville doctors and patients were heartened to see the dramatic benefit promin had on leprosy. But the medical community was cautious—other medicines had enjoyed the initial excitement of success and then proven disappointing. The careful clinical trials that are taken for granted today were not well developed then. An impassioned editorial in the *International Journal of Leprosy* in 1947 demanded, "This time, let's have the proof!"

The Fifth International Leprosy Congress, meeting in Havana in 1947, named sulfones the drug of choice, but reserved the possibility that other treatments might be superior. Within another year or two the international medical community was convinced. Ultimately one of the sulfones known as DDS, or dapsone, was found to be effective, relatively inexpensive, quite safe for most patients, and easy to use.

Dapsone soon became available to most of the world's patients around 1950, when transportation links were restored following World War II. Because dapsone works slowly, patients were instructed to take it for years—often for life. Its effectiveness, nevertheless, resulted in thousands of patients being discharged from leprosy hospitals and colonies around the world.

Finding a cure for an infectious disease is important and valuable, but a medicine that kills the bacilli in individual patients does not eliminate the disease from the population. Moreover, a cure alone leaves unanswered many questions, including: How is the germ transmitted? Why do some people catch it while others do not? Why do those infected with *M. leprae* develop so many different types of the disease? How do the nerves become injured, and can this be avoided? Can leprosy be prevented with a vaccine?

A major advance in growing *M. leprae* in the laboratory finally occurred in 1960, when Dr. Charles Shepard, working at the Centers for Disease Control in Atlanta, Georgia, succeeded in demonstrating limited but reproducible growth of this organism in the footpads of laboratory mice. The mouse-footpad technique was quickly adopted in major leprosy research laboratories around the world. At last a method was available to determine at least some of the basic information about the microbe itself, and to test new drugs in the laboratory. However, dozens (even hundreds) of mice are required for each test and, because *M. leprae* grows very slowly, each experiment takes nearly a year to complete. Such experiments are, therefore, both slow and expensive.

Several additional drugs effective against *M. leprae* have since been identified, due in part to the availability of the mouse-footpad technique. Combining two or three of these greatly improves treatment in individual patients and also greatly reduces the likelihood that the bacilli will become resistant to treatment. Use of these drugs in combinations is referred to as multidrug therapy (MDT).

Scientists working at Carville discovered another animal model in the 1970s. This one was literally in their back yard—the nine-banded armadillo. Although armadillos are larger and more difficult to maintain in the laboratory than mice, *M. leprae* produces an enormous number of bacilli in armadillos. Armadillos provided billions of bacilli for scientists throughout the world. With the number of bacilli available for research no longer a serious limiting factor, *M. leprae* could be subjected to the kinds of biochemical and immunological studies already well developed for other organisms.

This discovery led to another breakthrough, this one from the elegant biochemical studies conducted by Dr. Patrick Brennan at Colorado State University. Colorado, a state with only a few leprosy patients and no armadillos, was able to obtain large quantities of *M. leprae* from experimental armadillo colonies. This enabled Brennan and others to examine the outer wall of these bacilli, including the lipids and other chemicals in that wall that are the first components of *M. leprae* to be encountered by the cells of the immune system. Among the many substances they were able to purify, one of them, abbreviated PGL–1, appears to be unique to *M. leprae*. Several studies quickly determined that many leprosy patients make antibodies to PGL–1, and this offers the possibility that it may be used to develop laboratory tests for the diagnosis of leprosy. Research on this possibility continues.

Advances in molecular biology and genetics provide another way around the roadblock of noncultivation of *M. leprae*. Technical developments in molecular biology enabled scientists to determine the entire sequence of the DNA of this organism—its genome. This has made it possible to identify *M. leprae* using a technique known as polymerase chain reaction, or PCR. This method is now used to identify *M. leprae* and distinguish it from other organisms in unusual specimens or situations. The technique can also identify mutations that correspond with resistance to one or more of drugs used in the treatment of leprosy. There is also the possibility that by comparing portions of *M. leprae* DNA with that of other related organisms some genes may be found missing that are needed to culture it.

As already noted, clinical leprosy work and research have been guided since the mid-1960s by the realization that individual differences in immunologic responsiveness to *M. leprae* form

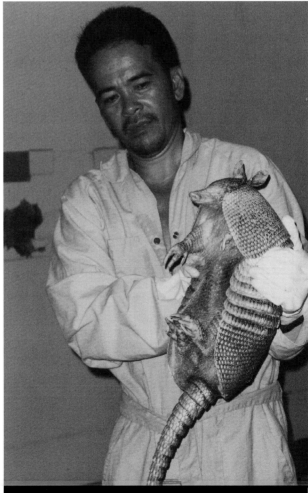

Armadillos have been instrumental in allowing the study of M. leprae *bacilli.*

On December 11, 1965, at the Ministry of Health of Ethiopia, the All Africa Leprosy and Rehabilitation Training Centre (ALERT) was legally established by representatives of five founding organizations: Orie O. Miller for American Leprosy Missions; A.D. Askew for the Leprosy Mission; Dr. Paul W. Brand for the International Society for the Rehabilitation of the Disabled; H. E. Ato Abebe Kebede, minister of public health; and Lij Kasse Woldemariam, president of Haile Selassi I University. The nucleus for the training unit was centered at the Princess Zenebework Hospital, built by the Sudan Interior Mission with funds supplied by ALM.

Miller reported that support from American Leprosy Missions called for:

a) Half support of Daniel Sensenig, seconded by the Eastern Mennonite Board of Missions to serve as business manager;

b) Full support of Dr. W. Felton Ross to become clinical director; and

c) Budgetary support for maintenance and capital of $125,000 over the next three years.

Other persons who contributed significantly to the early development of ALERT were Dr. Stanley Browne; Don McClure, treasurer of ALM; and Dr. Charles Leithead, chairman of the board and professor.

ALERT

The World Committee on Leprosy Rehabilitation, with Dr. Paul Brand as its chair, decided in a 1963 meeting in Carville that a training center should be created to focus on the rehabilitation of people affected by leprosy, particularly in Africa. Doctors Paul Brand and Stanley Browne were deputized to search for an appropriate location.

Addis Ababa, Ethiopia, was judged to best meet the criteria. An agreement was drawn up and signed in 1965 by the five founding organizations. The main goal of ALERT was "to train men and women in all aspects of leprosy with special emphasis on control, treatment and rehabilitation for work in African countries."

ALERT assumed responsibility for the existing Princess Zenebework Hospital and the new training and research facilities were gradually established there. The Armauer Hansen Research

Institute (AHRI) was inaugurated in 1970 on the same site, and has been closely linked with ALERT since.

The first director of ALERT was Major Onni Niskannen; Dr. Felton Ross served as the first director of training. Dan Sensenig was loaned by the Mennonite mission to serve as the first business manager. A number of donor agencies contributed significantly, including several from Scandinavia and members of the newly formed International Federation of Anti-Leprosy Associations (ILEP).

ALERT quickly became world renowned. From 1984 to 1999, 1,798 health care professionals received training there. Nine hundred eighty-two trainees were from thirty-three African countries (Ethiopia, 356; Nigeria, 203; and Tanzania, 69); 135 were from Asia (India, 29 and Pakistan, 15); and 681 trainees came from the rest of the world (the Netherlands, 237; Scandinavia, 165; Britain, 59; and U.S., 31).

In 1999, the 230-bed facility with an active outpatient department had a staff of 538, 5 of whom were expatriates. In that year there were 615 leprosy admissions. While the Government of Ethiopia supplied most of the personnel, operating costs were borne mostly by external donors, ILEP members, and Cristoffel Blindenmission (CBM) in particular.

ALERT continued to concentrate especially on leprosy-related research, advocacy, and the formation of people's organizations. With the declining prevalence of leprosy, however, interest in leprosy-only courses diminished. The trend in the 1990s was to combine leprosy and TB programs, resulting in changing the name to the All Africa Leprosy Tuberculosis and Rehabilitation Training Centre.

In recent years responsibility for leprosy and TB control activities was transferred to the Ethiopian Ministry of Health. Regrettably, it has not been possible for ALERT, the government of Ethiopia, and ILEP to agree on the legal status of ALERT; with the result that the program has been taken over by the government. How this will affect the service, training, and research activities remains to be seen. The hospital is presently busy, training activities are being maintained, and trainees continue to be sponsored by a variety of donors, including ILEP members.

—Dr. Paul Saunderson

the basis for many different manifestations of this disease. Discovering the mechanisms by which this works remains a major challenge in leprosy research. This work received great impetus from the explosion in knowledge about the immune system that began in the 1960s.

New methods made it possible to distinguish between different types of white blood cells called lymphocytes (which all looked similar using older methods). Lymphocytes provide specific guidance to the immune system. More recent work has identified the chemicals that they and other cells of the immune system use to communicate and direct the defense against *M. leprae* and other germs. These chemicals are called cytokines. As a result of other discoveries in basic immunology, biochemistry, and molecular biology, vanishingly small quantities of these can be measured and the activation of genes that produce them can also be identified.

All of this has enabled modern medical science to describe the immune response to *M. leprae* in very detailed manner, identifying the specific molecules being produced to control this infection. However, the results still do not explain how it is that most people seem to be naturally immune to leprosy, nor exactly how effective immunity to *M. leprae* can be stimulated.

A Vaccine?

This leads directly to one of the most frequently asked questions: Is a vaccine possible? This question has challenged many research programs since the 1960s, when details about immunity mechanisms in leprosy began to be deciphered. As noted, *M. leprae* is one of several germs and parasites that are not affected by the presence of antibodies. Consequently, the direct actions of immune cells are required. To date no vaccine has been developed that adequately induces strong cellular immunity against these organisms.

Intensive efforts were made in the 1970s to produce a vaccine. Included among those

attempting to produce a vaccine was an American, Dr. Barry Bloom. This initiative enjoyed substantial funding from the World Health Organization, as well as from the governments of several developed and developing countries. One approach was to use BCG, long used in the treatment of tuberculosis, although with limited effectiveness. Evaluation of a large field trial, also supported by the WHO, indicated a low level of protection, but insufficient to be of practical value for the treatment of leprosy.

In Venezuela, Dr. Jacinto Convit made a candidate vaccine using a combination of *M. leprae* and BCG, but after large-scale trials there and in Malawi, Africa, this also did not appear to be effective. Developing a vaccine able to induce effective, long-lasting cellular immunity is a major goal with potential benefits for many diseases, and so the effort continues. Currently, the most active research is an attempt to use

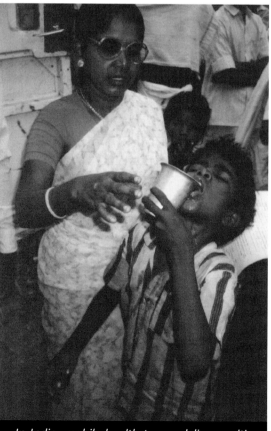

In India, mobile health teams deliver multi-drug therapy (MDT) to rural villages. Here, a child takes his MDT as neighbors look on.

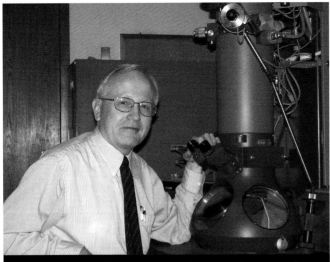

Dr. David Scollard using an electron microscope in his lab in Baton Rouge

DNA from the bacilli as a vaccine. This, too, is generating very interesting results in some experimental models, but a great deal of work is needed to determine its efficacy.

Finally, one sophisticated area of research at the beginning of this century focused on the question raised by Danielssen and Boeck more than 150 years ago: Is there a hereditary (genetic) influence on leprosy? We know that a germ causes leprosy, but abundant evidence now also clearly indicates that each of us inherits specific and sometimes limited capabilities to mount a defense against different diseases. Some genes may influence our ability to destroy *M. leprae* before infection can be established, and other genes determine how we will respond if the first line of defense fails. Revolutionary techniques developed in the 1990s allow geneticists to explore this subject in greater detail than could have ever been imagined even thirty years ago. The results anticipated in the next few years will undoubtedly influence the attempts to develop a vaccine.

Is Research on Leprosy Still Necessary?

Medical research is expensive and time consuming. But if progress in the age-old struggle against leprosy is to be made, research must continue. In contradiction to the impressions of some that basic research is abstract and impractical, it is this basic work that provides the foundation upon which the practical applications are built. It is hoped that the discoveries noted here by Hansen, Virchow, Faget, Doull and Guinto, Skinsnes, Ridley and Jopling, Shepard, Brennan, and others will prove convincing.

Medical science concentrates on questions remaining to be answered, not on what is already known. In leprosy, after over a century of study by some of the best and brightest medical scientists of each generation, many basic questions remain unanswered. Leprosy continues to challenge each new and more sophisticated technology.

The Task is Unfinished

- The total number of registered leprosy patients worldwide has dropped dramatically during the last twenty years, partly as a result of cures made possible by MDT. The total number of *new* diagnoses, however, has not declined and remains at about half a million annually. Why?

- Individual patients can be diagnosed and treated with a high degree of accuracy, but no vaccine is available to prevent leprosy. Can such a vaccine be developed?

- *M. leprae* is still not cultivable in a laboratory, and no simple, direct answer is available to the seminal question: How is this germ transmitted?

- The best means of early diagnosis is still a careful clinical examination by an experienced doctor, nurse, or health worker. Leprosy still cannot be detected until the infection is established, nor can it be determined if contacts such as family members have been infected. We must still do as physicians have done for more than one hundred years—watch and wait.

- The only laboratory tests available to determine if treatment is working are based on a biopsy, or "skin smear," and examined for bacilli, much as Hansen did in the 1870s. How injury occurs, and therefore how to develop specific means of treatment and prevention, is still not known.

This writing does not do justice to the patient and persistent efforts of hundreds of scientists from various nations on all continents over many generations. Nor does this account portray adequately the colorful character of the personalities that animate the story. This includes many extraordinary and engaging individuals who, with extraordinary dedication and self-sacrifice (some would say, stubbornness), are continuing to work to understand and solve the mysteries of this elusive disease.

ABOUT THE AUTHOR

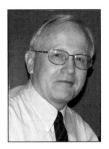

*D*avid Scollard is chief of research pathology for the National Hansen's Disease Programs, Baton Rouge, Louisiana, a position he has held since 1993. He is also editor of the International Journal of Leprosy. His primary research interests are the mechanisms of reactions and of nerve injury in leprosy.

Scollard was born and raised in North Dakota. He received a B.A. degree from St. Olaf College in Northfield, Minnesota, and M.D. and Ph.D. degrees from the University of Chicago. Before embarking on a career of leprosy-related research, he taught at the University of Hong Kong and later served as field director for an NIH-supported collaborative research project in Chiang Mai, Thailand. He has been a tenured member of the department of pathology at the University of Hawaii School of Medicine, and has published over fifty papers and chapters on subjects related to leprosy.

Scollard is married and has two children. He is an active member of St. James Episcopal Church in Baton Rouge.

Chapter 9

Rehabilitation: The Restoration of Dignity and Self-Worth

by Susan S. Renault

In 1993, then ALM president Thomas Frist had his design department create wall panels illustrating the effects of leprosy upon a "normal" person. Frist knew—and wanted his staff to know—that leprosy was not merely a medical complication. One illustration showed the psychosocial and economic decline many leprosy-affected people experience. This panel was called "Dehabilitation."

Dehabilitation is the undoing—the unraveling —of life. Dragged down by community fears, self-inflicted loathing, and ultimately a state of social, economic, and physical disability, the erect figure who once stood at the top of the scale tumbles towards the bottom and is finally shown bent and beaten.

The "Rehabilitation" panel illustrates the path back to normalcy. It is paved with a daunting assortment of obstacles. The poor fellow at the bottom can only reach the top through personal conviction, discipline, partnership-building, community education, medical intervention, and the goodwill of friends who believe as Tom Frist did that the multi-challenging path towards recovery does not end with a repaired hand or healed ulcer. It ends only when the man stands tall.

Tom Frist, Paul and Margaret Brand, Jean Watson, Hugh Cross, Linda Lehman, Jean Pierre Bréchet, Felton Ross, and legions of others— remind us through their own work, lives, and personal ministries that the ultimate goal of rehabilitation is the restoration of dignity. You

repair a hand so a man can work. But it's not about work; it's about worth. You restore a woman's face to its smooth almond color. But it's not about skin color; it's about dignity. You strengthen a teenager's foot so it will not drag when he walks. You are giddy when the surgery is successful. You've restored a boy's gait. You've restored hope.

Worth. Dignity. Hope. The words make the rehabilitation process seem almost poetic. Spiritual. These are the blessings God would want for all our lives. We "leprosy workers" are His hands; we are His servants. Our marching orders are clear.

The goal is simple, but the path is complicated. Our understanding of *how* to rehabilitate and *how* to restore dignity changes and grows. This very paragraph suggests a traditional view: How do *we* help *them* regain life?

The problem with we/them is sustainability. Anyone who has ever tried to lose weight, stop smoking, or become a nicer person knows that while the encouragement and empowerment of others is helpful, real change comes from a renewal of *your* spirit, a change in your own heart that moves you from "I can't" to "I can." Real recovery comes

Thomas Frist

when you have just the right balance of support, retraining, intervention, self-investment, and self-realization to move from "I can" to "I will." Ultimate success comes when "I will" becomes, "I will now; I will tomorrow; I will the day after; I will as long as I have life and breath. I will because I know my dignity is worth the effort. I choose to experience wholeness." Now *that's* a challenge!

It's a challenge that prompted Heather Currie and ALERT hospital colleagues in Ethiopia to initiate self-care groups in 1995 for the management of wounds. Traditional methods of hospital-directed soaking, oiling, scraping and dressing reinforced dependency upon hospital services and produced disappointing results.

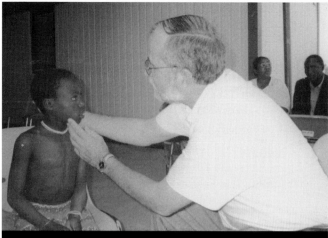

Mission doctor Jean Pierre Bréchet examines a child in Angola.

Self-care group membership was voluntary and open to those who wished to take responsibility for their own wound management. Members were required to come up with their own solutions for wound healing and their own materials for bandaging. They were given neither supplies nor money.

I visited one of these groups in Wolkeite in 1998. A dozen former leprosy patients sat in a circle. One person took a seat in the center of the group and held up his hands and feet for inspection. The peer review was thorough and critical. If a wound looked worse than last month, they criticized the care. One man had a cut finger that wasn't cut a month before.

"What happened?"

"I was sharpening a sickle."

"Next time, take it to the blacksmith."

"Yes, I promise. I will not sharpen it myself again."

Another man took the center seat.

"Your hands are dry. They will crack."

"Yes."

"Why haven't you been oiling them?"

"I can't afford the oil."

Other groups discussed ways this man could earn money for petroleum jelly or oil, then rendered their verdict: "If you get desperate," they told him, "sell your jacket. Your hands are more valuable than your jacket!"

The next man came to the center of the circle. He had no wounds. His feet were clean and ulcer free. The group celebrated with a round of applause.

I noticed that many of the wounds were bandaged with fibrous strips of material, and I learned the group had discovered a most ingenious alternative to cloth (hospital-supplied) bandages. They had torn cellulose strips from the stems of the false banana leaf. Their new bandages were sterile, molded easily around the limb, were plentiful, and were free! According to an article by Benbow and Tamiru, "At first, some of the members were reluctant to use these strips because they were considered to be a *traditional* material, but following the wound healing results of others using false banana bandages, they changed their minds and began to use them."

Benbow and Tamiru cite a number of unexpected outcomes from the self-care group program and quote group members:

- "We participate in society now. For example when we attend a coffee ceremony, we don't hide our hands and feet anymore. . . ."

- "We don't go to the hospital or orthopedic workshop for ulcer treatment any more. Why should we? We can do it ourselves."

- "Because we no longer smell and are surrounded by flies, my daughter married into a non-leprosy family."

- "Once we were dependent on the hospital and had wounds; now we are independent and we don't have wounds because we can heal them ourselves; now we have our dignity and self respect."

What this group demonstrated, and what rehab specialists like Jean Watson, Hugh Cross, Catherine Benbow, and others have long understood, is that membership in an effective self-care group has benefits that extend beyond wound management. Members of the group learn to minimize deformity-producing complications; in turn this makes possible their inclusion in their larger community group.

This is not only true in Ethiopia. In a September 2001 *Leprosy Review* article on ulcer prevention, Cross wrote about community dynamics in India. "In the Indian subcontinent there is no strong concept of 'self.' It is the corporate need of the body of the family (closely followed by the need of the community) that is significant rather than the individual in isolation. Accordingly, when individuals are denied a role in the family and community their lives are perceived as essentially meaningless. Effective ulcer management enables a person to continue as a member of his community; unsightly deformities often spell the end of group acceptance and membership."

It's not skin patches that people equate with leprosy; it's deformities. Lalgadh Hospital in Janakpur, Nepal, goes to great efforts to include self-care training in every aspect of rehabilitation (and, thus, preserve group status). Patients practice hand and foot exercises, self-care techniques for farming activities, self-care for kitchen tasks, and a variety of other POID (prevention of impairment and disability) for daily activities.

One of the simplest self-care adjustments I witnessed was in a model kitchen. The simple

Care After Cure

In 1986 a special study on care after cure was initiated at Karigiri hospital in South India. Sponsored by the Baptist Union of Sweden, the study identified and cared for the medical, rehabilitative, and socio-economic needs of patients who had completed their treatment and yet were unable to fend for themselves because of deformities. This was an important study as it highlighted the fact that care was very different from cure.

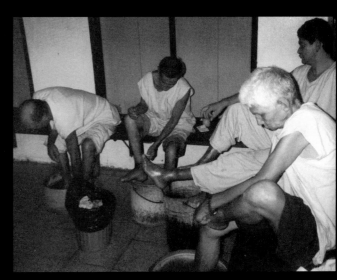

Bathing ulcerated feet

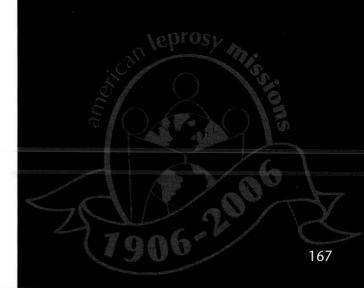

mud-like structure is designed to look and feel like the kitchen women will return to after they complete their self-care training. A woman was sitting on the hard floor, holding a round, tray-like basket and winnowing rice. Her feet were curled up underneath her. She tossed the grain into the air, separating grain from chaff, and repeated the procedure several times. Then she stopped, remembering something important. She put the basket down, pulled over a short wooden stool not more than a couple inches high, hoisted herself onto the stool, and resumed her work. Her work triggered a message that went something like this, I'm speculating: "If I raise myself off of my legs and ankles, I'll relieve pressure and possible skin breakdown; if I relieve pressure, I'll decrease the risk of wounds and ulcers; if I decrease wounds and ulcers, I have a better chance of being allowed back into my community."

This small, wooden stool, integrated into the total rehabilitation program, was a powerful ingredient in the rice winnower's recipe for successful wound-management. And, like other self-care graduates, she would leave Lalgadh with an understanding of the personal responsibility and skills to manage a life with leprosy.

Sustainability

The issue of sustainability drives the orthopedic staff at Green Pastures Hospital in Pokhara, Nepal. Stand in the shoe and appliance workshop and you'll see very little stainless steel. You won't hear the whir of precision Swedish instruments or be awed by German technology. What you will see are competent technicians—craftsmen, almost—whose artistic hands shape leather, plaster, and nuts and bolts from the village market into custom-fitted shoes and braces. This is no amateur operation: the folks here are serving patients with spinal cord injuries; babies with club feet; mothers with broken necks; teenagers with leprosy. Serving, restoring, rehabilitating.

I visited the GPH workshop in 2003, and couldn't help thinking: *I might be able to get a donation from such and such bio-technology company. Or, maybe I could get a grant for the latest and greatest mechanical devices.* I wanted to take a well-functioning, technology-appropriate, patient-empowering, sustainable workshop, and turn it into the Mayo Clinic. I couldn't help myself. I'm still a recovering "we/they" thinker.

Hugh Cross shared a story about a man in China who lost both legs below the knees, and illustrated patient-appropriate technology. He was shuffling about on his knees but was getting wounded. So he cut up car tires to protect himself. He found if he cut more tire than just what he needed for knee protection, he could improve his method of movement. He cut about a third of a tire for each leg, padded it to protect himself, and then inserted his knees and lower legs into the tires. This left a significant segment of the tire going out in front of him. The tires gave him a roll forward movement rather than just staggering from stump to stump. He actually had quite a good rolling motion while also protecting his knees from damage. He solved his problem himself.

Says Cross, "It really is quite wonderful the way people adapt when there is no help at hand. Indeed, I sometimes feel that it is better not to make adaptations for people because they may not be sustainable. If people can do their own problem solving and be creative with the resources they have, it is far better."

Catherine Benbow has a similar tire story about a man she met in East Timor:

The man had recurrent ulcers. He had made his own sandals from rubber tires and

Hugh Cross

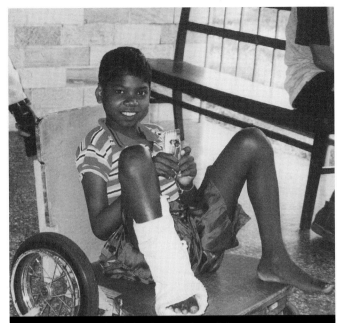

Dumka received both hand and foot surgery at ALM-assisted Green Pastures Hospital in Nepal.

flip-flops shaped to minimize pressure on his wounds. The man understood biomechanics though a carpenter by trade. I realized without any doubt that . . . I needed to work with them, to encourage them and only share what I had learned if it made sense to them. When I told this man that there was another man with terrible ulcers just over the hill, he immediately offered to go and see him. In my heart and mind, that was the beginning of the self-care group idea.

Nearly all the rehab specialists I spoke with have systems they've developed for sustainable care. Jean Watson eschews pharmaceutical eyewashes and drops for many people with leprosy-related eye problems. "I find it is unrealistic in rural China to obtain supplies of artificial tears for life. Even to splash what should be clean, boiled water onto the eyes is rarely feasible."

Watson prefers instead the self-disciplined, patient-motivated "trigger therapy." Certain agreed upon triggers remind people to do a single, strong blink. "I teach clients the effort that *they* need to make to cover the cornea, repeated at intervals during the day and on the triggers." Typical triggers are a passing vehicle, a farmer winnowing, the sight of blowing dust, wind on your face, walking past a house, and walking past a tree. In Nepal, Watson says, patients learn to exert special effort to close their eyes each time they greet one another with the customary "namaste" greeting.

Watson credits Dr. Margaret Brand with developing the original "think blink" concept. Her own multiple trigger system is a variation on Brand's system of encouraging thirty blinks at each meal.

Self-care, whether for eyes, hands, or feet, is a lofty ideal. "Younger, newer patients are more likely to comply," Watson says. "Older patients who have had lagophalmos for years are less likely to comply until their eyes become uncomfortable."

So how do *we* get *them* to understand the benefits of self-care? How do *we* get *them* to begin the daunting climb back up the rehabilitation path? How can *we* get *them* to blink their eyes and protect working hands from catastrophic injury and to reshape habits to minimize injury and maximize normality? How do *we* get *them* to care?

Developmental experts like Matthew Maury (ALM director of community-based ministries, 1999–2002) believe the answers lie in CBR, community-based rehabilitation. People need a stake in their rehabilitation efforts. It's the WIIFM principle: "What's in it for me?"

Maury was zealous in his mission to convert traditional we/they thinkers. He brought fresh insights into the dynamics of change. Like Frist, he operated from the premise that dignity is rarely conferred upon one person by another; it comes because people engage in social efforts that recognize the mutual value, worth, and intelligence of all participants. Experts learn to relinquish power, control, decision-making, and program direction to the real stake-holders. This can be hard on experts. They must revise their expectations and agree to accept the needs which the community group identifies. It's not just the experts, though, who must shift paradigms.

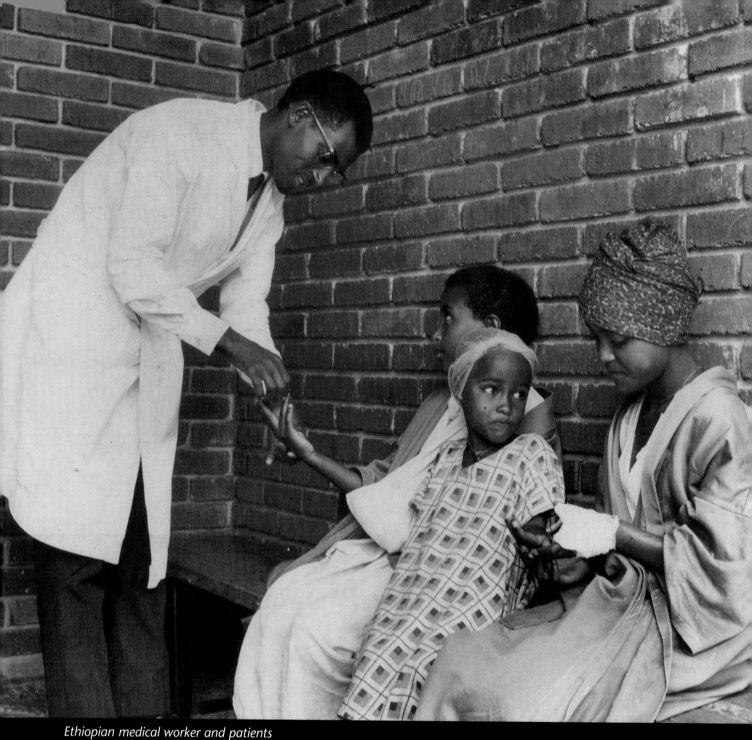

Ethiopian medical worker and patients

Long-term leprosy clients frequently resist the CBR approach. The person who has lived an entire life being cared for may not wish to break this dynamic. CBR is hard work!

By the time Maury left ALM to return to Habitat for Humanity in South Africa, many ALM project partners embraced some form of CBR. ILEP members and WHO are including CBR in their integrated approach to rehabilitation for people affected by leprosy.

In a June 2002 dialogue paper published by American Leprosy Missions, Maury offered a useful definition of CBR by Einar Helander (*Prejudice and Dignity: An Introduction to Community-Based Rehabilitation* [New York: UNDP, 2002] 8).

Community-based rehabilitation is a common-sense strategy for enhancing the quality of life of people with disabilities by improving service delivery in order to reach all in need by providing more equitable opportunities and by promoting and protecting their rights. *CBR builds on the full and coordinated involvement of people with disabilities and their families.* (chapter author's emphasis)

One of my favorite CBR experiences comes, again, from Ethiopia. The settlement that has developed around the periphery of the ALERT hospital is one of the largest leprosy colonies in the world. To the visitor, it is a haphazard and frightening collection of teetering boards, rickety posts, and shaky foundations. Crowded shanties compete for space along muddy roads and perilous potholes. Make a list of every conceivable social ill that comes from impoverished ghetto life and you'll come up with a description of the leprosy village. Life is harsh for old people; it holds little promise for the young.

It is here that Sister Senkenesh Mariam heads the Medhen Social Centre, a ministry of compassion and restoration. In the late 1990s, in the spirit of CBR, Sister Senkenesh invited her neighbors to voice their most urgent need. The community obviously needed better roads, clean water, medical care, and access to jobs, but the parents spoke loudest: "Our children's education is poor. If they are ever to escape the stigma and poverty of the leprosy village, they must have better skills."

"How would you get teachers?"

"We will engage our older children, the ones who have completed some schooling, to become tutors for the younger ones."

"What will you use for classrooms?"

"We will build them."

When I visited the tutoring centers in 1998, children crowded eagerly around their tutors to recite their letters and review their lessons. They sat in the shade of humble shelters, erected by gnarled and fingerless hands— erected without benefit of modern tools. I thought about the signs: "Road under construction," "Children under construction," or, perhaps better yet, "Futures under construction."

Is Life Really Sacred?

I suggest that the Christian view is that the unique thing about human life is the spirit, that is, the means by which we know God. The physical body of a man is just the framework. It remains the same as any other living tissue, yet it can be the temple of the Holy Spirit . . .

My specialty of rehabilitation brings me into close contact with quadriplegics and other disabled persons whose disease has cut them off from most of the means of self-expression and most of the life they enjoyed before their disease or accident restricted them. I often have had the feeling that a spirit is struggling to grow and longing to reach out and express itself in love; but it is frustrated by weakness, or by the attitudes of others towards the physical deformity by which the spirit is confined. The opportunity to work with such a spirit and help to free it is one of the most inspiring challenges open to us. No effort is too great and no expense should be spared to restore activity to such a one or to help the spirit to rise above its physical limitations and witness to the Grace of God whose strength is made perfect in weakness. Thus, even the most grossly disabled and diseased individual is dignified and made a worthy object of devotion and care by the fact that he is the home of the spirit and is actually, or potentially, in the image of God.

—**Paul W. Brand**
in "Is Life Really Sacred,"
published by The Christian
Medical Fellowship, London, 1973

If the children of Ethiopia are under construction, some of the adults have achieved a status never even imagined in their younger, sadder leprosy-focused days. One of the most memorable people I met in Addis Ababa was Ato Arega Kassa. He had multiple deformities and, I believe, a prosthetic leg. I recall he was nearly blind.

His bearing suggested victor more than victim. He was garrulous and likable. Despite bad eyes, hands, feet, and most every other part that showed, he conveyed strength and dignity. He told me he was planning to attend an international leprosy meeting in another country. I nodded politely as a parent would for a child who announces she'll become president some day—kind of a "that's nice, dear," response. After all, how could a maimed old fellow, blind to boot, possibly navigate the rigors of overseas travel? The idea seemed preposterous.

Of course, such an idea would have been preposterous years ago. How could a deformed person expect to enjoy the freedoms and privileges of "normal" people?

The answer was IDEA (see page 192), an international leprosy self-help organization composed of leprosy survivors. Ato Arega was president of the Ethiopian chapter. He practically *glowed* with a sense of well-being. He was a man with a mission, and his life would no longer be defined by his disease.

Dr. Yo Yuasa, past president of ILA, spoke about the founding of IDEA as follows:

> It is a great achievement indeed, though long overdue, to create such an organization by, of, and for the persons affected by Hansen's disease. I am particularly happy as well as impressed to note that the basic stance of the association is totally forward looking rather than backward glancing. You are not asking us to remember and to compensate for a terrible fate the members of your association have suffered in the past, but asking us to join hands as equal partners to build a society in which, whatever the physical condition, each individual is able to live with dignity as a human being and that life is integrated fully into the society.

No discussion of rehabilitation is complete without a round of applause for Anwei Skinsnes Law and others of like mind. Anwei had the craziest visions of people with leprosy traveling to leprosy congresses and international forums—*of participating in their own restoration and reclaiming the dignity they'd lost along with their fingers and toes*. In 2001, IDEA sponsored the first International Conference on Issues Facing Women Affected by Leprosy held in Seneca Falls, New York.

No discussion of CBR, POD, sustainability, appropriate technology, self-care, and holistic rehabilitation is complete without paying tribute to the giants who paved the way for specialists like Lehman, Benbow, Winslow, Watson, Bell-Krotoski, Piefer, Wim Brandsma, and others.

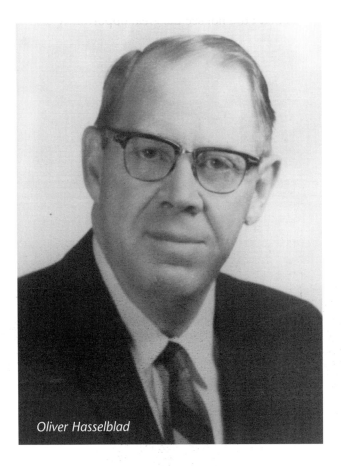

Oliver Hasselblad

Ask these experts who inspired them and you'll probably hear the same names: Paul and Margaret Brand, Frank Duerksen, Ernest Fritschi, and Oliver Hasselblad. These are the pioneers whose surgical techniques, teaching gifts, and godly spirits made young people say, "That's what I want to do. I want to be like them."

Surgeon Frank Duerksen read about Dr. Paul Brand in the condensed book section of *Readers Digest* before he started medical school. He was intrigued by Brand's pioneering hand surgery, and a dream was planted. As a child, Duerksen visited the Km. 81 hospital in Paraguay. He knew at age seven that he wanted to become a physician; Dr. Schmidt at Km. 81 often talked about Duerksen someday working at the busy Mennonite hospital. "I just laughed," Duerksen said.

In medical school, his textbook devoted one and a half pages to leprosy.

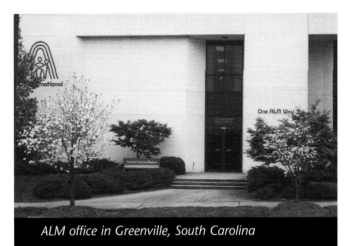

ALM office in Greenville, South Carolina

> After that, I told Dr. Schmidt that I would not dedicate my life to a disease that could be described in one and a half pages.

> Then something happened out of my control. In 1968, I was in a surgical residency in Bs. Aires . . . Dr. Schmidt wrote letting me know it was their year of furlough to go to the United States. Clara and their children had already left. He could not leave, because the doctor that was supposed to replace him had become seriously ill and would not come. He asked if I would come and help?

Duerksen declined. Then a second and more urgent letter arrived from Schmidt: "You have to come or else I will not see my family for a year!" Duerksen finally agreed. After all, treating a disease that takes one and a half pages and getting paid for it didn't sound half bad.

> When we arrived at Km. 81, I had to rush to the delivery room to deal with a difficult birthing, and the work seldom stopped for the four months we were there. I had to treat hundreds of leprosy patients in the hospital as well as in the rural control program. My one and a half pages was not enough to even start to understand this complex disease . . . I noticed the nerve lesions, especially the hands. But at this point my connection to leprosy surgery was still far away. General surgery, obstetrics, reactions and neuritis, foot ulcers, amputations, etc. overloaded me so that I did not see the great opportunity of my life, to combine missionary work with hand surgery.

> That connection came later in Winnipeg when I received a letter from Dr. Paul Brand from Carville and a ticket to come and visit him for a weekend. Dr. Hasselblad from ALM would also be present. My stomach stretched to my ankles! Dr. Paul Brand, *the Dr. Paul Brand,* would like to see me! Would I come? I flew higher than the airplane.

> Dr. Brand and Dr. Hasselblad explained the need for a surgeon to be located in South America with the purpose of training surgeons and rehab teams for leprosy . . . "Would you be willing to train for a year with Dr. Ernest Fritschi (at ALERT) and then return to South America?" *It was at this moment that my eyes were opened to the unlimited hand surgery to be done.* I said yes and the rest is history.

Dr. Fritschi could not get the visa for Ethiopia, so Dr. Paul Brand came twice to teach me. I had the master all to myself! At the end of my year, Dr. Fritschi arrived. He left his suitcases and operated non-stop for a week to transmit his knowledge. So I had two masters as my teachers.

Dr. Hasselblad taught me more about leprosy and leprosy rehabilitation. But definitely Dr. Brand, through his life story and his direct interacting with me, was the stronger factor.

(*Author's note:* I have heard it said, "Nearly all the good hand surgeons in South America today received their training from Dr. Duerksen." Not a bad legacy for a student who began with reservations about a "one-and-a-half-page disease.")

Another tribute from Catherine Benbow:

I was totally fascinated by the reconstructive hand surgery Paul Brand pioneered, which is not surprising since I was working as a hand therapist in the UK. It was his story and his work that made me want to do leprosy-related work, plus the testimony of one of his students, Mary Verghese. Paul Brand thought like an Occupational Therapist (so I could relate to him) because his aim was to promote improved functional independence for the individual, whether footwear, working with tools, self care, employment, community participation and spiritual well being. He paid attention to detail.

Benbow was inspired by Jean Watson as well.

When I realized that nerve function loss could be reversed if diagnosed early, it was the enthusiasm of Jean Watson that inspired me to work with field staff to develop good techniques to determine muscle weakness, feeling loss, and nerve tenderness and to prescribe additional medication. There is nothing more wonderful than to see the expression on a patient's face when he says, "It is normal again. I can work again and feed my family. I can feel."

Paul and Margaret Brand are also on Linda Lehman's list of mentors. "They demonstrated and pursued excellence but never forgot the importance of relationships," the ALM disability-prevention specialist said. One of the Brands's endearing qualities (Lehman also found this in Felton Ross and Ruth Winslow) was their willingness to listen . . . and to share their time.

(*Author's note:* Lehman learned well from the masters, and is, herself, a sensitive listener and loving encourager.)

In his chapter on stigma, Hugh Cross quoted the late Professor Valencia of the Philippines: *"The disease is perceived as one that uglifies not only the body but the soul; it turns, though slowly, a person into a thing."* We paraphrase that to read as follows: *"Rehabilitation is that which beautifies not only the body, but the spirit; it turns, though slowly, a thing into a child of God."*

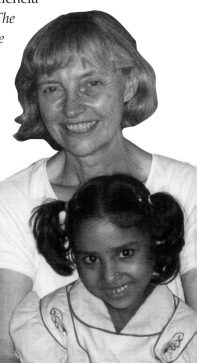

Susan Renault with girl in Nepal

ABOUT THE AUTHOR

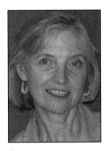 *Susan S. Renault is ALM's director of communications. During her fifteen-year tenure, Renault has made extensive visits to ALM-supported projects. In 2000, the Greenville Chapter of Women in Communications named her professional communicator of the year; and in 2002 she won a first-place Matrix Award for a direct mail package she created. Renault is a graduate of Northeastern University in Boston, and took graduate classes at the American Graduate School for International Management in Glendale, Arizona.*

Renault is married to Lance, chief program officer at ALM, and has two grown children. She is active at John Knox Presbyterian Church in Greenville, where she teaches adult Sunday School, sings in the choir, and is moderator of Presbyterian Women (PW).

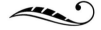

Chapter 10

Leprosy Plus

by Christopher J. Doyle

Leprosy registers are shrinking. On a global level, the number of cases has been reduced to less than one per ten thousand population (1:10,000) in the year 2004. Leprosy treatment is increasingly being integrated into general health programs. "Horizontal" treatment is replacing the old "vertical" model. The World Health Organization is poised to announce that leprosy has been globally eliminated as a public health problem. Much of what leprosy workers have long hoped and prayed for has been realized.

Welcome as this news is, ALM field reports show that the number of new cases waiting to be discovered and treated continues unabated. Leprosy remains a serious public health problem in at least fifteen countries. Chief among them is India, which has the world's largest leprosy population. The scourge of stigma is still an everyday reality, crippling leprosy-affected people even after the germs are destroyed. Clearly, ALM and other anti-leprosy agencies know their work is not finished.

This confronts ALM with the challenge of reinventing itself. In so doing it has studied the experience of other agencies including the March of Dimes, whose mission was originally narrowly focused on the treatment of polio. When a vaccine was discovered, its leaders knew that for the March of Dimes to remain viable, it had to broaden its focus from polio to birth defects. This involved adjusting its programs and reeducating its supporters. It did just that, and today the March of Dimes continues to be a successful and needed charity.

Similarly, ALM went about studying new ways to use its expertise and resources. Its leaders reminded themselves that MDT alone does not restore health and dignity. It is naïve to say, "Just take your medicine and everything will be all right." Patients who have completed their MDT continue to experience discrimination and marginalization. MDT kills the bacteria but not the stigma. ALM leaders resolved that as long as there were children and families in need, ALM would stay in the "leprosy business."

This led ALM to broaden its focus to include other debilitating and stigmatizing diseases and to move from cure to care with a focus that includes non-leprosy neighbors and communities. Cure was redefined to include the resulting disabilities. From these studies and discussions emerged what has increasingly become known as "Leprosy Plus" or "CurePLUS."

Disability Prevention

The sad truth is that despite the good work ALM and colleague agencies have done to cure leprosy, people continue to damage nerve-deadened limbs and eyes rendered insensitive to pain by leprosy. As long as fingers are worn away and feet are wrapped in bloody bandages, leprosy-affected persons will not gain acceptance in their communities. Injuries lead to disability and poverty. Injuries cause stigma.

POD Consultants

In 2001 ALM strengthened its global technical presence by engaging two regional POD consultants, Dr. Hugh Cross and Linda Lehman. Dr. Cross is based in the Philippines and is a teaching, monitoring, and evaluation resource to ALM project partners in Asia. He is a podiatrist with extensive third world experience in the prevention and management of leprosy-related disabilities. Linda Lehman is based in Brazil and serves in the same capacity as Dr. Cross but in South American and Africa. She is an occupational therapist with advanced training in the management of the hands and feet problems many experience, especially in Brazil.

As ALM's leprosy work shifts to a stronger emphasis on the prevention and management of disabilities, we need to provide more technical back stopping to our project partners. This means teaching project partners and patients about POD, advocating the integration of POD into national leprosy control programs, monitoring the care provided to patients, and conducting periodic evaluations of ALM funded projects.

Although our two regional POD consultants are specialists in the prevention and management of leprosy-related disabilities, they are dedicated to a holistic approach to the treatment and care of people affected by leprosy. They are quite knowledgeable in the medical and socio-economic aspects of leprosy, and in this capacity, they provide an important additional level of project oversight between Greenville-based staff and our project partners. These two regional positions insure that our project partners are trained and are using all the necessary skills to bring health and wholeness to people affected by leprosy.

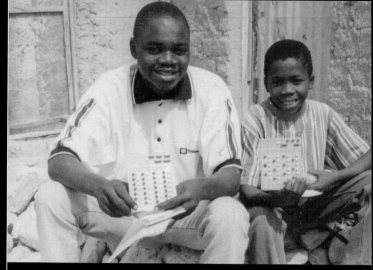

Young boys hold the blister packs which contain MDT drugs cure their leprosy.

Leprosy Plus embraces services beyond the "find and cure" strategies ALM has traditionally followed. These services include POD, the Prevention of Disability. In 2001, ALM's Brazil specialist, Linda Lehman, became a fulltime POD consultant, overseeing programs in South America and Africa. Hugh Cross was appointed POD consultant for Asia.

Lehman recalls a landmark meeting with the ministry of health in Brazil in 1986 that established a model of POD work integrated with MDT.

> Dr. Maria Leide knew that leprosy could not be treated with drugs alone. Some critics felt she was too slow and cautious about MDT distribution, but she was introducing a comprehensive program that did far more than kill bacilli. This partnership resulted in integrating MDT, POD and rehabilitation in a holistic control program. Because of Leide's influence, POD was an integral part of Brazil's general leprosy control program.

According to Lehman, one of the stars of this meeting, and of the early days of leprosy control work in Brazil, was Dr. Felton Ross. "Many people in Brazil owe their training to him. He wouldn't let them forget the nerves!" Another significant supporter of holistic care was Dr. Frank Duerksen, who regularly left his practice in Canada to teach surgery in Brazil and Paraguay.

Thus, ALM has a legacy of seeing "cure" as only a *part* of a much bigger emphasis that addresses nerve damage, disability, and even social issues.

Holistic Services

Health workers continue to face the challenge of normalizing lives, engaging community support for leprosy-affected people, and supporting grassroots efforts to empower individuals educationally, economically, medically, financially, and spiritually. Much work remains to be done to achieve the second part of ALM's mission statement: "To be a channel of Christ's love to people with leprosy and disabilities, helping them to be healed in body and restored to lives of dignity within their communities."

Leprosy Plus involves equipping leprosy-affected individuals and communities to live normal lives. This means moving beyond twelve doses of MDT to encouraging community-based initiatives that affect general health, literacy, hygiene, economy, and spiritual growth.

The Jamkhed, India programs serve as a model. Begun many years ago by the Arole family, the program seeks to enable people to pursue lives of dignity within their communities. Through community-based initiatives and program development, leprosy-affected people at Jamkhed become community leaders and health workers. They replace stigma with strength and helplessness with resolve.

Early in the year 2000, ALM's Program Department sought collaboration with selected international non-profit organizations. Their search led to partnership arrangements with agencies like Habitat for Humanity International, Heifer Project, and other governmental and non-government organizations. Through these partnerships, leprosy-affected families are helped to realize lives of dignity within their communities. They are able to build houses, raise livestock, and make a living through small-business ventures. Partnerships with church and mission agencies increase ALM's ability to provide spiritual discipleship and Christian nurturing.

ALM has reaffirmed in this century its commitment to Christ-centered, people-based, and sustainable, holistic ministries. Its programs are need-based and participatory. They are culturally relevant, collaborative, and developmental

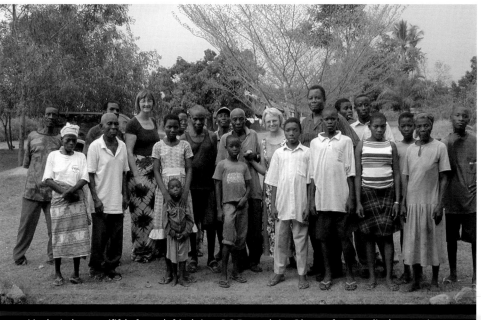

Linda Lehman (fifth from left) doing POD work in Ghana for Buruli ulcer patients

The Mission of ALM Reiterated

The soft-spoken, British accented admonition of Dr. Margaret Brand to the ALM board was: "Even one case of leprosy is significant to the person who has it." Dr. Brand continually reminded people that "Before our work is about reaching goals and targets, this ministry is about people. Individuals tend to get lost in big initiatives and audacious goals. It is up to the leprosy charities to keep the focus where it should be, on people."

2002 International Leprosy Congress

At the International Leprosy Congress, held in Salvador, Bahia, Brazil in August 2002, the ILA issued the following statement:

> The ILA General Meeting of Members wishes to make it clear that the available evidence strongly suggests that a significant leprosy problem will continue to exist for many years to come and that services to detect and manage cases of leprosy must therefore be sustained. The ILA General Meeting of Members calls on all stakeholders (including national governments, international organizations and non-governmental organizations) to review their recommendations and guidelines for leprosy-related activities. . . .

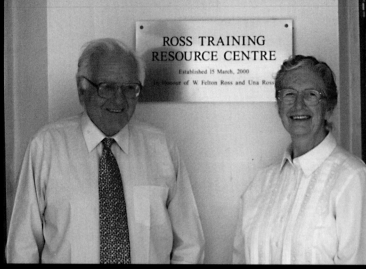

Felton and Una Ross at the dedication of the Ross Training Center at ALERT

instead of charity oriented. Preference is given to programs that are environmentally sound, gender sensitive, and inclusive.

In 2004, ALM introduced a Cure*PLUS* campaign in the *Word & Deed* newsletter as part of its reeducation effort. Every gift of $240 provides the services to cure *and care for* a person with leprosy. "The cure kills the bacilli," donors are told, "but it is only the beginning of the restoration. ALM believes God wants to complete each troubled life. Cure alone does not pave the way to a future of promise and possibility, but Cure*PLUS* does."

Treating Other Diseases

The most obvious question that faced ALM in its effort to expanding its ministry to other diseases was *which other diseases*? Spirited discussions marked ALM board meetings. Staff engaged in brainstorming and debate. Eventually, a consensus emerged:

- Treat diseases similar to leprosy. This similarity may be genetic such as tuberculosis, or it may be similar in how it damages the body, such as Buruli ulcer, which devastates whole communities in West Africa. These diseases and health problems can be treated with the same staff and facilities, and sometimes with the same drugs.

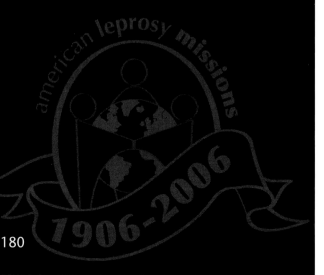

- Treat "orphan diseases," ignored by most international organizations. These diseases do not make headlines nor do advocacy groups, celebrities, or lobbyists publicize their plight. Marketing orphan diseases is obviously a huge challenge. Who, after all, has heard of lymphatic filariasis and leishmaniasis, even though millions suffer their ravages?

- Treat diseases that stigmatize. One of the lessons of the past one hundred years is that loneliness, rejection, isolation, loathing, and abuse are more painful than ulcerated toes. People who carry the double burden of disease and stigma are the very people who need most to experience Christ's love. ALM continues to feel called by God to offer a comforting hand to "the least of these."

- Treat diseases that prey on children. By finding them in the earliest stages maiming, heartache, and stigma can be minimized.

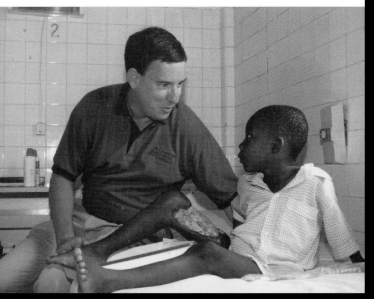

ALM's "other disease" is Buruli ulcer, a flesh-destroying disease that attacks mostly children under the age of fifteen. Buruli is a public health problem in Ghana and Ivory Coast. Here, ALM's Christopher Doyle visits with a young patient.

Out of the Corner

Living in South India, leprosy left him with stumpy fingers and a broken spirit. Health workers concluded that his cure was incomplete even though he had finished a regimen of MDT. To help him become economically self sufficient, he was given a small loan with which he bought four bicycles to open a rental business. With hard work he was able to buy two additional bicycles and start a repair shop. Visitors watched incredulously as he wrestled a stubborn tire from the rim with the almost fingerless hands with which he has literally pulled himself out of poverty.

After some years Srinivasan was able to qualify for a housing loan, satisfying that important need in his life. His emotional and economic recovery lifted him to a position of respect within his community. "He no longer sleeps all day in the corner," reported his family. Had his treatment ended with the last dose of medicine, this proud man might have slept his life away in some dark corner, never discovering the joys that God had in store for him.

Major Trends in the Treatment of Leprosy

The last twenty years leading to ALM's centennial celebration have seen the most significant advances in the treatment and care of people affected by leprosy. This was led by WHO's approval in 1981 of MDT as the treatment of choice. Three major groups have been instrumental in bringing about the successes we have witnessed:

1. The World Health Organization (WHO) has provided a global awareness and call to action through:

   A. the creation of a specialized leprosy unit within the Communicable Diseases Group and a Technical Advisory Group (TAG) for leprosy elimination;

   B. the strong advocacy for leprosy elimination among the leprosy endemic countries;

   C. the establishment of leprosy elimination targets for endemic countries;

   D. the advocacy of case detection campaigns and simplified field diagnosis; and

   E. a key logistical role in the supply of MDT.

2. Government leprosy services in endemic countries became proactive with:

   A. the creation of broad-based national leprosy control programs using MDT;

   B. the integration of specialized leprosy treatment services into general health at the peripheral level of public health services;

   C. the transition from institution-based treatment and care of routine cases to outpatient treatment and care;

   D. the conversion of specialized leprosy hospitals into general hospitals; and

   E. the integration of POD (Prevention of Disabilities) services in major national programs as an integral part of the leprosy diagnosis and treatment regimen.

3. Non-government organizations (NGOs) such as ALM led the way in the international financial and technical support of government programs as well as the development, advocacy, and provision of services not included in many government programs. These include:

   A. supplementary funding for government and NGO treatment and care programs at all levels in endemic countries;

   B. international leadership in the professionalization and expansion of leprosy-related disability prevention and management, with an emphasis on self-care;

   C. developing community-based rehabilitation models in partnership with people affected by leprosy;

D. the advocacy and implementation of socio-economic assistance for people affected by leprosy;

E. the subsidizing of anti-leprosy drugs by the Novartis Foundation and the Nippon Foundation; and

F. developing service delivery networks between non-leprosy-specific NGOs and leprosy-specific NGOs, for a more holistic approach to restoring people affected by leprosy.

The bottom line to these efforts has been twenty years of continuing improvement in the treatment and care of people affected by leprosy. We have joyfully witnessed:

- earlier case detection, which means less disability right from the start;

- the rapid and permanent cure of the disease with MDT;

- prompt and effective management of complications that may occur;

- better strategies in all aspects of treatment and care to help those disabled by leprosy; and

- more effective measures to combat stigma and discrimination against people affected by leprosy.

—**Lance Renault**

In short, each new Leprosy Plus initiative should be a logical outgrowth of ALM's century of treating leprosy.

As a result, in the year 2000, the ALM board agreed to expand its agenda to include victims of Buruli ulcer, a flesh-destroying disease that preys mostly on children and is most common in Ghana and Ivory Coast, West Africa. Every bit as devastating as leprosy, victims are often treated cruelly and, like leprosy, as objects of stigma.

This historic decision was inspired largely by medical consultant and past board member, Dr. Wayne Meyers. A former medical missionary in Africa, Meyers spent more than two decades studying Buruli ulcer and its effects. He spoke passionately about the disease most board members had never heard of. "The expense, disability, isolation, and rejection BU victims face is akin to what leprosy-affected people have endured for generations," Meyers told the board. "The wounds penetrate body and spirit."

ALM found already established, compatible project partners in Ivory Coast and Ghana to administer this expanded ministry. While broadening its focus to Leprosy Plus, ALM continued to make leprosy its first priority.

Beyond Leprosy Plus: A Vaccine

In November, 1999, American Leprosy Missions boldly adopted as its vision statement: *Christ's servants, freeing the world of leprosy.* Simply ministering to people with leprosy, as many have done for more than a century, is not sufficient. ALM is not satisfied to *reduce* leprosy. The vision is to free the world of this scourge.

No disease, history tells us, has been eliminated without a vaccine. MDT, for all its good, cannot complete the task. Before anti-leprosy organizations can consider their work completed they need to make one final push to answer questions that have stymied medical workers for ages: How is leprosy transmitted?

How can it be determined who is susceptible and who is not? How can leprosy be prevented? In the words of Professor Cairns Smith, international renowned leprologist, "We cannot eliminate leprosy with what is known today. We must know more." This calls for research.

Leprosy research has, in fact, decreased decidedly since the discovery of MDT, as there was premature optimism that it would accomplish eradication. In the meanwhile, research has led to the mapping of the genome for leprosy and scientists are able to picture the leprosy bacillus. Mapping the genome was a huge leap forward, but still short of the mark.

Against this background, after years of debate and with the strong advocacy of board member Dr. John Dawson, the ALM board determined in the year 2000 to make a final assault against *M. leprae* by launching a $7 million campaign to invent a leprosy vaccine. The Infectious Disease Research Institute (IDRI) in Seattle, Washington, joined ALM in this ambitious endeavor.

Efforts are underway to identify specific proteins of *M. leprae*, using the recently published description of its genome. Such proteins may additionally have use as new diagnostic agents that may allow earlier diagnosis of infection. These twin tracks are being pursued vigorously.

ALM projects in DR Congo provide curePLUS. For example, the projects may provide cure plus a fishing net or cure plus house repairs. In this photo, the boy on the left has leprosy. ALM donations are paying for his school fees, as well.

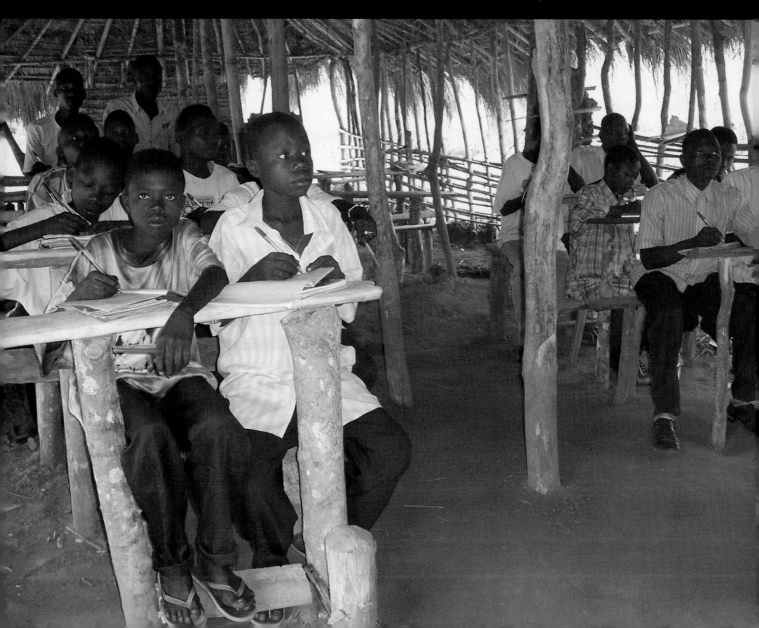

Nippon Foundation and the Sasakawa Memorial Health Foundation

Within the family of agencies associated with ILEP is the influential Sasakawa Memorial Health Foundation (SMHF) and its parent agency, the Nippon Foundation of Japan. The Nippon Foundation began its program to eliminate leprosy in 1974 with the establishment of the Sasakawa Memorial Health Foundation. Though that organization has since branched into many other fields, its principal objective was, and remains, the elimination of leprosy.

When the World Health Organization (WHO) officially recognized MDT as a cure for the disease, the Nippon Foundation's Yohei Sasakawa pledged enough money to provide treatment for all patients everywhere of every country. During 1995–1999, WHO provided all MDT drugs, free of cost, to nearly eighty countries utilizing a fifty-plus-million-dollar drug fund donated by the Nippon Foundation.

The SMHF provides funding and technical advice to the WHO leprosy unit, national leprosy control programs, and various NGO leprosy programs around the world. Dr. Yo Yuasa, medical director and executive director of SMHF, and Dr. Felton Ross, medical director for ALM, shared a lasting friendship built on mutual professional respect and commitment to the Christian faith. ALM and other agencies fighting leprosy could not have had the impact they did without the provision of free drugs by the Nippon Foundation and the facilitating and implementing role of SMHF.

In the twenty-first century, the Nippon Foundation, working through SMHF, announced a pledge to contribute twenty-four million dollars to WHO to assist in the implementation of a global leprosy elimination strategy.

—Lance Renault

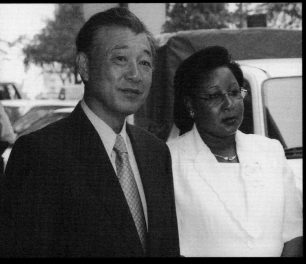

The Nippon Foundation's chairman Yohei Sasakawa has made control of leprosy his life's work. In 2004, he was named WHO Goodwill Ambassador for Leprosy Elimination. He's pictured here with Albertina Julia Hamukuya, Angola's minister of health.

IDRI, it is encouraging to note, has already had notable success in using this same approach with both tuberculosis and leishmaniasis.

It is with a deep sense of satisfaction and gratitude that ALM reflects on a century of work in behalf of those afflicted by one of the world's oldest and most tragic diseases. Much has been accomplished; multitudes have experience healing and hope.

As we celebrate the past we scan the horizon and are humbled to realize that our task is not completed. Facing us are new opportunities to spread Christ's message of redemption and compassion wherever He leads us.

ABOUT THE AUTHOR

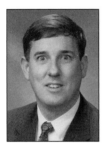

Christopher J. Doyle became president and chief executive officer of American Leprosy Missions in 1995. Under his leadership, and with the growing success of MDT, ALM's programs have expanded beyond cure to care after cure and to the treatment of other debilitating and stigmatizing diseases.

Doyle has served on ILEP standing committees and action groups and on the boards of the Schieffelin Leprosy Research & Training Center in Karigiri, India, and the Leprosy Mission Trust, India.

He is a member of Christian Management Association and also serves on the board of Evangelical Council for Financial Accountability. Doyle's articles about fundraising and non-profit administration have appeared in Christian Management Report, The Star, *and various ILEP publications.*

A graduate from Columbia International University in Columbia, South Carolina, Doyle and his wife, Karen, have four children. They are active at Mitchell Road Presbyterian Church, PCA, in Greenville, South Carolina.

Chapter 11

Peering into the Future

by Paul Saunderson

As ALM reaches its centenary, there is an incredible explosion of biomedical knowledge and research. This is having an effect on almost every human disease, as well as broader biological problems facing humankind. Decoding of the genomes of a whole range of organisms—from human beings to the leprosy bacillus—brings hope of breathtaking advances in the control and treatment of infectious disease and in the prevention and management of cancer and other non-communicable diseases. These new technologies, assisted by advances in computer science, are developing so rapidly that the future is difficult to predict. Most poignantly for our purposes: Can leprosy be eradicated? Is eradication a worthy goal?

The future of leprosy cannot be discussed in isolation from other considerations, including the issue of poverty, since leprosy is a disease of the poor. It is transmitted particularly amongst the poor and it impoverishes its victims. While headline-making international conferences discuss global poverty reduction, many countries are poorer at the beginning of the twenty-first century than they were a decade or two ago. Their weak health systems cannot provide the level of care needed for common diseases including leprosy. Private clinics everywhere provide sophisticated medical care for the rich, but the masses are less fortunate. What real hope is there that the poor will benefit from the biomedical advances in the next few decades?

The question facing ALM and its colleague agencies is how it should invest its energies. Making eradication the goal is obviously expensive and the outcome uncertain. Some are inclined therefore to opt for *managing* leprosy, just like any other disease. Give new cases the best treatment available, they argue, thus reducing disability and deformity; work to reduce stigma through community education programs. Management, not eradication.

Others argue that however expensive the development of new tools and vaccines, failure to utilize them will result in unnecessary disability that will in the long run be more costly, to say nothing of the needless suffering involved.

ALM believes both approaches should be pursued, since no one can know which strategy will achieve the greatest good. Aggressive and systematic case finding along with quality patient care and self-care must continue while the search for better technologies continues. If tools to accomplish eradication, which our predecessors have longed for and fervently prayed for, are now within reach, ALM intends to use them and participate in their development.

Leprosy Control and Treatment

The first hundred years of ALM's existence can be divided into two roughly equal parts from the viewpoint of leprosy control.

During the first fifty years, up until around 1950, the only way to control the spread of this infectious disease was to isolate those affected, although there was vigorous debate over the practicality of this policy. In practice, it led to much suffering, as families were separated—even newborn babies were separated from their mothers, supposedly for their own protection.

Isolation was pursued with varying degrees of vigor. In Norway, for example, a tolerant policy allowed patients to live at home, but they had to be segregated within the home, living in different rooms. In some countries, the policy was harsher; while in others isolation was considered of little value and not practiced at all.

During the second fifty years, antibiotics changed the outlook for people affected by leprosy. Cure was possible and it was quickly realized that antibiotics rendered patients non-infectious, making isolation unnecessary. Unfortu-nately, it took years for this to be accepted by policy makers and the general public.

Multidrug therapy (MDT) brought with it the possibility of cutting the chain of transmission between patients and their contacts. This raised hope that the disease could be eradicated.

One of the most important determinants of eradication is the absence of an animal reservoir. If a disease is present in animals, it is not considered eradicable. If, on the other hand, the disease only exists in humans, as was the case with smallpox, and as is the case with polio and lymphatic filariasis, eradication may be possible. It is not entirely clear how this applies to leprosy since it has been found in some animals such as armadillos in southern United States. There is no evidence that an animal reservoir is important in maintaining leprosy in the human population.

Eradication of leprosy is possible if transmission can be cut. MDT was introduced globally during the 1980s. The results were impressive. Unfortunately, by the year 2000, it was clear that transmission was not being reduced as hoped.

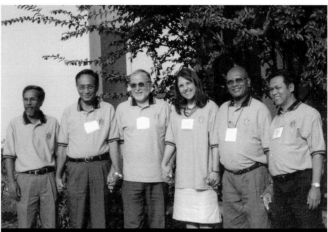

ALM Field Reps (left to right): F. Thomas Mathew (India); Dr. Tim Shane (Burma); Dr. Jean Pierre Bréchet (Angola); Dr. Zoica Bakirtzief (Brazil); Dr. Jacques Kongawi (DRC); and Randy Pepito (Philippines)

The number of new cases detected remained stubbornly high and, more important, new cases in children remained static.

The leprosy incubation period is variable—typically from three to eight years or more. But for children it obviously cannot be longer than their life span. Thus, if MDT has been effectively implemented in a country for more than fifteen years and the number of children under fifteen diagnosed with leprosy remains unchanged, it is axiomatic that transmission is continuing.

Why MDT has not stopped the transmission of leprosy is not known, but the most likely explanation is that transmission occurs early during the course of the disease, before the diagnosis is made and MDT treatment is started. The incubation period may be very long—as much as twenty years—and towards the end of that period a patient may be transmitting the infection before signs or symptoms appear. Even after the first signs appear, patients may not immediately seek help because the early symptoms are mild—just a few skin patches that do not seem troublesome.

As ALM celebrates its centenary, one overwhelming challenge is to find strategies to interrupt transmission of the disease. Only then can the eradication of leprosy be considered possible.

A Three-Pronged Approach

Three different approaches may help to interrupt the transmission of leprosy. It may be possible to use them in combination, achieving even greater effect. They are as follows:

1. *New diagnostic tools:* Methods to detect leprosy infection early during the incubation period, before the disease is passed on to contacts. Through early detection, treatment can be immediate and transmission greatly reduced.

2. *Chemoprophylaxis:* Treat populations most at risk of getting leprosy (perhaps through contact with another leprosy patient) and thus prevent infection. The medication (possibly a single dose of rifampicin) is safe and relatively inexpensive, so treating people who would not end up being infected is not a major problem; the main question at present is whether a cost-effective and feasible chemoprophylactic strategy can be developed.

3. *Vaccine development:* Develop a vaccine that will induce lasting immunity. An ideal vaccine will boost the body's defenses and thus fight off leprosy at any stage. If someone already has leprosy, a vaccine can be therapeutic and cure the disease. If leprosy is in the incubation stage, it can be stopped and cured without reaching the symptomatic stage. If the person is not yet infected, future infection is prevented.

ALM is utilizing all three approaches. The main objective is, of course, to find an effective way of interrupting transmission. Each approach may also provide other benefits, making each investment doubly worthwhile. The most obvious additional benefit of early treatment is the reduction of nerve damage and disability.

Definitions

Definitions from the WHO International Classification of Functioning, Disability and Health:

Deformity is a visible impairment.

Disability is an umbrella term, used in a rather broad sense.

Impairments are problems in body function or structure.

Activity is the execution of a task or action by an individual.

Activity limitations are difficulties an individual may have in executing activities.

Participation is involvement in a life situation.

Participation restrictions are problems an individual may experience in involvement in life situations.

Stigma means "a mark," indicating disgrace or disrepute. Its use is often extended to mean the social exclusion associated with a certain condition, such as leprosy, AIDS, or mental illness.

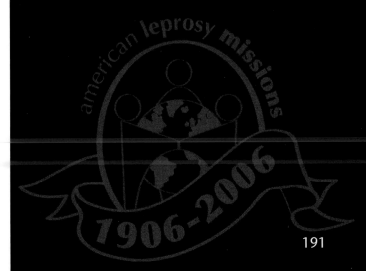

Chemoprophylaxis is being studied in Bangladesh in a Leprosy Mission research project largely funded by ALM. It is not likely that all people at risk can be identified; but even if a proportion of cases can be prevented, it will be worthwhile. They will be spared physical damage or social isolation that still affects many patients. As many as 30 percent to 70 percent of cases could be prevented, depending on local conditions. Here are some of the questions that need to be answered in the next five to ten years:

- Can a fairly small group of people at greater risk of developing leprosy be identified?

- Can leprosy be effectively prevented in this group with a simple treatment?

- What proportion of all new cases can be prevented in this way?

- What is the most cost-effective way of organizing such a program?

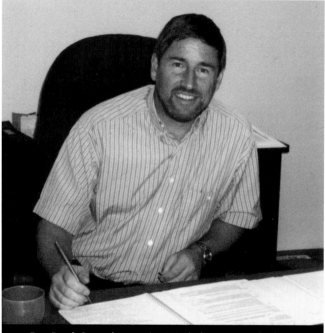

Dr. Paul Saunderson is ALM's leprosy consultant and medical expert. He joined the staff in 2000.

There is some evidence that as the amount of leprosy in a community decreases, new cases are more likely to be found in households of already known cases. This means that as the incidence of leprosy declines, strategies of chemoprophylactic treatment of contacts may be increasingly effective and lead to a decline in transmission.

The field of new diagnostic tools is complex. While there are methods of directly detecting the organism, they are generally cumbersome and require expensive equipment. Indirect methods, which could be used in ordinary clinics, are generally based on detecting the immune response of the body. There are two types of responses and until now, it has been assumed that two separate tests will be needed.

Many leprosy patients have a relatively mild infection because they have a strong natural resistance to the disease. They are termed "paucibacillary," or "PB," cases, from the Greek meaning "few bacilli." Effective resistance to leprosy comes about through cell-mediated immunity (CMI), in which T-cells directly engulf and destroy the leprosy bacilli. Few antibodies are produced.

Other patients with little natural resistance have a heavy infection. They are termed "multibacillary," or "MB," cases, from the Greek meaning "many bacilli." These patients do not show much CMI, but they do produce antibodies that, unfortunately, do not seem to provide any protection. In PB cases, CMI could be detected by skin tests like the one used in tuberculosis. In MB cases, skin tests are negative, but antibody tests are generally positive.

An added complication—and why such tests are not yet in routine use—is that normal people who do not have leprosy frequently test positive on one or other of the available tests. This is thought to be caused by bacteria in the environment that are quite similar to leprosy and that many people are exposed and become immune to them, causing a cross-reaction.

What are needed are skin and antibody tests that are highly specific—that only read positive when leprosy is actually present. With publication of the leprosy genome and other advances in antigen discovery, improved diagnostic tests can be developed based on a few well-defined proteins. They may be used initially in research studies to gain a better understanding of the epidemiology of leprosy, especially at the community level. This may help to target chemo-prophylaxis more accurately and make it more effective—an example of the benefits of combining these several approaches.

It is hoped that one or more highly sensitive and specific diagnostic tests will be available within two to three years.

ALM is supporting the development of new diagnostic tools indirectly. The ALM Centennial Vaccine Campaign also involves antigen discovery. The same basic laboratory studies will provide the groundwork for both new diagnostic tools and potential vaccines. While a candidate vaccine may be available for trials in about five years, it may take a further ten years of field-testing to establish its usefulness.

By using a combination of the three approaches mentioned, it may be possible over the next decade to develop new, more effective strategies for leprosy control. If transmission of leprosy can be reduced globally during the following decade, and more or less stopped by 2030, it is possible that new cases of leprosy would no longer appear after about 2040. The number of new cases appearing in the two decades between 2020 and 2040 could be very low, if the methods to reduce transmission also prevent disease effectively in those already incubating it. People who have had leprosy and who may have some leprosy-related disabilities will have a normal lifespan. Therefore, with increasing longevity, it is certain that some people with leprosy-related disabilities will still be alive in the year 2100.

This projection is relatively conservative; some steps may proceed more quickly. Nerve damage, for example, may be more effectively prevented, bringing about a more rapid reduction in permanent damage. On the other hand, it is also possible that unseen obstacles will slow progress and that leprosy will linger in poorer communities longer than expected. Certainly, even today many children still develop severe, permanent nerve damage because of leprosy.

A potential obstacle is the cost of implementing new measures on a global scale. Disputes over cost-effectiveness may conclude that some new tools are not useful. One way of controlling costs is to keep leprosy research closely linked to tuberculosis. Many control strategies are the same for both diseases, and if vaccines for both diseases can be given together or combined into one vaccine, significant savings may be possible.

New Treatment Regimens

In marked contrast to tuberculosis, the fight against leprosy is not hampered by a lack of effective antibiotics. There are new drugs available, which have not been introduced on a large scale because there is no need for them at the moment. Rifampicin remains a highly effective and very safe drug, and because it is more than thirty years old, it is now relatively cheap. MDT has, as of now, almost completely eluded drug resistance, so the basic drugs continue to be effective universally. This is one of the great successes of MDT.

As already mentioned, early diagnosis is the main challenge, and once the diagnosis is established, there is very little difficulty in ridding the body of the infection. It does not seem likely that new antibiotics will be developed that are significantly more effective than rifampicin, although a vaccine may have the effect of allowing a shorter course of treatment. Such advances, which may allow one regimen for all

IDEA: International Association for Integration, Dignity, and Economic Advancement of People Affected by Leprosy

Established in 1994, IDEA is the first international advocacy organization whose leadership is largely made up of individuals who have personally experienced the challenges of leprosy, also called Hansen's disease. With more than thirty thousand members in thirty countries worldwide, IDEA works as an agent of social change.

IDEA seeks to end the social isolation that is often associated with leprosy. Social isolation can be felt in the middle of a big city or on a remote island. It is experienced by individuals who are newly diagnosed and reluctant to tell their families they have the disease. It is also experienced by members of the older generation, who have lived most of their lives in physical isolation and, due to rapidly declining numbers, often feel more alone than ever.

Just as better ways of measuring physical disability are being developed, so the measurement of social exclusion and stigma is being addressed, leading to the development of more effective interventions. Such interventions can address society in general to help change attitudes towards those with disability, including those affected by leprosy. Other interventions are needed to help individuals deal with their own specific situation. Often the shame felt by someone with leprosy is the biggest obstacle to normal participation in society.

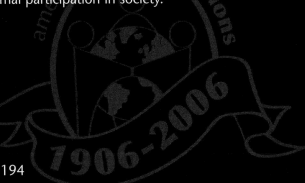

cases and a significantly shorter course, would be very helpful in the logistics of leprosy control.

Possibilities in Genetic Research

The decoding and greater understanding of the genomes of many organisms, including the leprosy bacillus and *Homo sapiens,* could potentially result in new diagnostic tools and treatment strategies contributing to eradication.

What is just as exciting, although perhaps more remote, is the discovery of individual genetic differences (that is differences between individual human beings), which may eventually explain why most people never get leprosy (even if exposed) and why, amongst those who do, some develop more serious complications than others. The immune system is complex and under the control of an array of genes. It is becoming clear that susceptibility to infectious diseases, as well as many non-communicable diseases, is influenced by an individual's genetic make-up. Perhaps not surprisingly, our knowledge in this area is most developed in the field of HIV/AIDS. At least one gene, found in only a small percentage of the general population, is almost fully protective against HIV infection. Such knowledge can lead to a better understanding of the pathogenesis of each disease, and perhaps then to novel methods of treatment and prevention.

Not only may some factors leading to infection be identified, but also the ways in which reactions and neuritis occur will become more clearly understood. This will provide another avenue through which complications may be better controlled. It is foreseeable that in twenty years a genetic screening test will be available that will indicate the likelihood of complications of leprosy developing and allow preventive measures to be taken.

Here too, as always, there is the barrier of cost. Research is very expensive and tools and resulting technologies are likely to be out of the reach of the people for whom they are intended.

Preventing Impairment, Disability, and Isolation

Efforts to prevent or reverse impairments in leprosy are another key area of interest for ALM, as is physical rehabilitation (although it is important to remember that many, perhaps the majority of people with leprosy-related residual impairments, neither need nor desire any form of therapeutic intervention to "rehabilitate" them. What occupies their attention is their place and role in society and in the local economy). Finally, we examine what is often referred to as socio-economic rehabilitation (SER), seeking ways of restoring people to lives of dignity within their communities.

The complete eradication of leprosy (no transmission and no new cases) is certainly a worthy goal; whether it is achievable in this century, either from a technical or an economic point of view, is unknown. Meanwhile, however, many people continue to suffer its consequences.

It is important to realize that the mutilating and deforming effect of leprosy is not due directly to the bacillus itself, but rather to the immune response of the body to the presence of the bacillus, or even the remains of dead bacilli. This means that even when effective antibiotics have been administered and all the bacilli are dead, new nerve damage may still occur, with devastating results.

For example, an impairment may appear minor and have no effect on activity (for example, loss of eyebrows in leprosy), but because of stigma and the reaction of other people, may lead to significant social restrictions. An impairment may appear severe (for example, amputation of a limb) and lead to some activity limitations, but participation may not be restricted if a good prosthesis allows more or less normal mobility and there is no stigma.

Psychological states, such as depression or anxiety, which may be precipitated by a medical problem like leprosy, are impairments that may lead to varying degrees of activity limitation and participation restriction. Medical problems can have grave economic effects, perhaps through loss of work, and this may have a major effect on participation.

This terminology is very helpful when one considers intervention options: medical interventions tend to be aimed at repairing or reversing the impairment itself and physical rehabilitation deals especially with minimizing the degree of activity limitation, while counseling and socio-economic rehabilitation focus on restoring participation.

There are a number of impairments that are typical of leprosy that may lead to activity limitation. Impairments and activity limitations may lead to participation restrictions for physical reasons (someone who cannot run cannot participate in a game of football), but also—and perhaps more important—for psychological reasons: someone with leprosy may not be invited to community events such as weddings or funerals, or if invited, may be too ashamed to attend (self-stigma).

Preventing Impairments

The typical signs of disability and deformity are caused by the predilection of the bacillus for the peripheral nerves. In biopsy material, bacilli may be found in the skin, but they are usually seen in larger numbers in the peripheral nerves, where they invade and live in the Schwann cells. Schwann cells are those that nurture and protect the neurons, the cells actually carrying and transmitting nerve impulses. When Schwann cells are damaged, the neurons lose their ability to function properly and eventually die.

Current research is beginning to explain the mechanisms by which *M. leprae* enters the Schwann cell, but it is not clear how much damage the bacillus itself does. Most damage seems to occur as a result of leprosy reactions, in which the immune system overreacts to the presence of the bacillus (or even to bits of long-dead bacilli still present) and damages the Schwann cell in the process.

Leprosy Reactions and Their Management

Leprosy reactions are complex events in which inflammation occurs in the skin and/or the peripheral nerves. If the nerves are involved, loss of function may occur, resulting in loss of feeling and/or paralysis of the muscles. Because the leprosy bacillus favors cooler parts of the body, it is the nerves in the limbs and around the face that are most affected, determining the characteristic patterns of nerve damage seen in leprosy. Because the eyes, hands, and feet are so important for daily activities, impairments frequently have severe consequences—both activity limitation and participation restriction.

Mild cases of inflammation in leprosy reactions can be treated with aspirin, but if nerve function has been affected, steroids are used to reduce edema and reverse the underlying inflammatory process. It is generally assumed that if the loss of nerve function has been present for six months or more, much of it will be permanent; if, on the other hand, the condition is recognized and treated in time, full function can be restored in 60 to 80 percent of cases. It is important, therefore, that front-line health workers know how to recognize and manage these reactions effectively so unnecessary suffering can be avoided.

By far the most important way to prevent nerve damage, as already stated, is early diagnosis and treatment. Drugs such as azathiaprine and cyclosporin are being tested to see if results can be achieved with fewer side effects than with steroids. The severity of nerve damage varies, and if the inflammatory process is prolonged or keeps recurring, the likelihood of permanent nerve damage increases.

Will it be possible to prevent reactions and nerve damage altogether, even if infection with the leprosy bacillus occurs? A recent study examined the use of prophylactic steroids to reduce the risk of subsequent nerve damage; the results were disappointing. Although there was less nerve damage initially, after twelve months there was very little difference between the treated and the non-treated groups.

More aggressive protocols may be able to prevent reactions and nerve damage through better understanding of the underlying mechanism of reactions, or because they can be more specifically targeted. Similarly, if the mechanism by which *M. leprae* enters the Schwann cell can be elucidated, it may be possible to design drugs which will interfere with the process and greatly reduce the numbers of bacilli that remain in or near the nerves. If that could be done, reactions may be much less dangerous, since the nerves would be less involved in the inflammatory process.

Again, funding is the limiting factor. New drug development is extremely expensive and it seems doubtful that any new and sophisticated drug targeted at one aspect of leprosy will be pursued to completion. It seems likely that new drugs will only be developed for more lucrative markets and any benefit for leprosy patients will be coincidental.

Another area in which new drugs may have an impact is the regeneration of damaged nerves. There is already evidence that some recovery in nerve function may occur naturally. If this can be speeded up or made more complete, many leprosy-disabled persons will be helped.

It is to be anticipated, therefore, that there will continue to be a gradual improvement in the diagnosis and management of reactions and nerve function impairment. This may be helped by new screening tests, but it will also depend on the knowledge, skill, experience, and dedication of thousands of front-line health workers in endemic countries. The challenge, particularly as the number of cases declines, will be to make these new technologies and the skills needed to deploy them available at the point of need.

Physical Rehabilitation

People with permanent leprosy-related impairments (loss of sensation, muscle weakness, or deformities of hands and feet), will be around at least until the end of the twenty-first century, although by then in very small numbers, adding to the challenge of serving them. Not all those with residual impairments need or want any form of rehabilitation, although an important minority can be greatly helped by appropriate therapy. This emphasizes the importance of a proper assessment of each individual, so the right assistance is offered. Demand for rehabilitation is complex and may increase as societies become more developed—not only are the services more accessible and of better quality, but people with disability may be more aware of the different options open to them.

The assessment of activity limitation in a standardized way is in its infancy, but great strides are in the offing. Future patients will be more accurately assessed, so that specific interventions can be targeted to their needs. ALM staff and funds helped to develop the so-called SALSA assessment tool (Screening Activity Limitation and Safety Awareness), which is in the

In D.R. Congo, Mayoyo has "dropped foot" and will injure his feet and toes without protection. Dr. Jacques Kongawi, right, has brought new shoes to Mayoyo. The shoes will be equipped with a small strap that lifts the foot when Mayoyo walks.

The P-scale: A Scale to Measure Participation Restriction in People Affected by Leprosy

An international, multi-center research project has developed a standardized questionnaire which can be used to assess the degree to which a person is isolated and unable to participate in normal community activities. This questionnaire can be used to compare the experience of people affected by leprosy in different communities and also to compare experiences over time, for example, before and after a particular intervention. In this way, the interventions to reduce stigma can be evaluated and improved.

As the "poorest of the poor," people affected by leprosy usually only make progress economically when development is community-wide. Many ALM partners have a commitment to holistic development—attending to every aspect of community life, not just health or disability. A basic element in this approach is the empowerment of members of the community so that ownership of projects and activities, and the accompanying decision-making authority, can be transferred.

The Millennium Development Goals are targets for poverty reduction and development over the next fifteen years. They are ambitious and will require concerted effort by governments, international bodies, and non-governmental organizations. It is very difficult to predict what sort of progress will be made in these areas, as so many factors are involved. Community-wide gains will help people affected by leprosy look after their own needs better, provided there is little stigma.

form of a questionnaire, enabling rehabilitation workers to quickly identify problems in carrying out everyday activities.

Available interventions include physical and occupational therapy (perhaps including various types of assistive and protective aids to improve function and minimize damage), as well as surgery, implants, and prostheses to minimize activity limitation. Appropriate footwear can prevent damage in people with loss of sensation on the sole of the foot. Although some are best helped by specially made shoes, shaped to a particular individual's feet, most do very well with mass-produced soft shoes now being sold quite cheaply in the most remote marketplaces. Everyone affected by leprosy should have access to the footwear he or she needs.

Great strides have been made in managing the eye complications of leprosy. It is important that such services are made available to those needing them. Even now, most problems that present are not due to leprosy, but to other common conditions, such as cataracts in the elderly. This illustrates the principle that people with leprosy will greatly benefit by all forms of community development targeted at the poor, including the improvement of general health services.

A significant change in the field of rehabilitation is the transition from institutional care and service to community-based rehabilitation (CBR). There is a great deal of discussion about how this concept should be worked out in practice, how it should be organized, and how it will be financed. The potential for more effective and more accessible care exists.

Perhaps one of the most important underlying goals is the empowerment of people—all people everywhere—in permitting them to participate in their treatment decisions.

Many people with residual impairments from leprosy are now members of self-help groups that, through mutual support and better access to information and other resources, enable them to cope more effectively with the consequences of the disease. This goes well beyond what can be achieved by a top-down, medical approach, in which an expert technician "rehabilitates" a more or less passive patient.

Economic Empowerment and Community Development

One of the most distressing aspects of leprosy is the stigma and social isolation that affects many to varying degrees. This very frequently leads to unemployment and severe economic hardship. A need for advocacy continues, seeking to reverse the prejudice that lurks under the surface in so many communities.

People affected by leprosy need practical support to gain access to the training and jobs they require to achieve their rightful place in society. This is beginning to be seen as a human rights issue, so that discrimination because of leprosy will become less acceptable and even unlawful.

Integration

Leprosy used to have its own separate health system in many societies—because of stigma, people with leprosy could not attend normal clinics and hospitals. In recent years this separation of services has almost disappeared, and leprosy work is being integrated into the general health services.

It is expected that all aspects of the health services in poorer countries will become increasingly integrated, so that local clinics will serve as the gateway to expertise on a wide range of fields and specialties. This should make it easier for anyone with leprosy to get the best treatment available. The danger is that if leprosy is rare in a certain community, health workers will not recognize it in time and patients will be diagnosed very late, as happens also in the western world. Modern technology (for example, tele-medicine, in which details of a case, including pictures, are sent to a consultant miles away) could be harnessed to make useful information more readily available.

Training of Physiotherapists (PT) and Occupational Therapists (OT) at Karigiri

In the past, only a few dedicated individuals were willing to sacrifice a "normal" career to work with people affected by leprosy. In the recent years, however, large numbers of PT and OT students in South India colleges have come to Karigiri for a short period of training. They find it challenging to learn the basics of leprosy and get experience with typical problems faced by people along with a range of other disabilities. Some conclude their studies with a short internship.

There is presently no universally accepted way of funding health care, so affordability remains a barrier for the poor. It is a significant achievement (through the leadership of WHO and others) that the basic treatment for leprosy is free of charge to everyone who needs it. There are, of course, significant costs in training staff, running clinics, case-finding, etc., but these costs are not passed on to the patients.

Training

As leprosy prevalence diminishes, the challenge to give health staff at various levels enough training to maintain an adequate service increases. What is needed is the ability to access the necessary information easily and on a timely basis, whether in printed or electronic form. Training needs to help people to solve the problems they encounter in their work.

As rehabilitation activities become a more significant component of leprosy control, helping people to live normal lives, a wider range of professionals must participate.

Leprosy is thus becoming part of the basic curriculum for a greater number of trainees and is being seen as an interesting disease. It has much to teach us about rehabilitation, but is not essentially different from many other conditions.

Conclusion

The dawn of the twenty-first century has seen amazing developments in biomedical science. The impact is enormous and still unfolding. Perhaps the biggest uncertainty is not over technology but affordability.

More immediately, leprosy workers everywhere are buoyed by evidence that leprosy is beginning to be seen as a normal disease, like any other complex condition. Reactions and neuritis are medical problems that can be very rewarding for clinicians to treat. With free treatment offered in integrated clinics, patients can enter through the front door, rather than being seen in a hovel behind the clinic with a separate entrance. This is a tremendous step forward. People affected by leprosy now have increased options and can be active in planning for their own future.

As we peer into the future we are humbled by the realization that we now have many of the tools our predecessors lacked. We enjoy what was the object of their fervent prayers. Whereas they were limited to care, and they did it with such compassion, we have the potential to cure victims of this dreaded disease. Beyond care and cure, we are participating in their rehabilitation. No longer are they banished and despised, they are able to live useful and productive lives.

Still missing is the ability to prevent leprosy from preying on future generations. This too, in God's loving providence, is now within reach and is part of the unfinished agenda we take with us as we enter our second centennial, seeking still to be Christ's servants, freeing the world of leprosy.

ABOUT THE AUTHOR

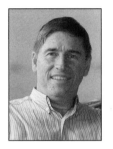

Dr. Paul Saunderson has been ALM's leprosy consultant since 2000. Originally from Cambridge, England where he trained as a physician, Saunderson spent almost twenty years in Africa, first in a remote mission hospital in Uganda administering the national leprosy and tuberculosis control program. In Ethiopia, Saunderson worked at the All Africa Leprosy, Tuberculosis and Rehabilitation Training Centre (ALERT).

Saunderson has served on numerous advisory bodies, including ILEP's Technical Commission and WHO's Technical Advisory Group. He additionally serves as honorary treasurer of the International Leprosy Association.

Saunderson has been involved with a variety of leprosy-related research projects, resulting in more than thirty scientific publications. His thesis on the epidemiology of nerve damage in leprosy gained him a doctorate at Cambridge University, England. He has also contributed to training materials published by ILEP.

Saunderson is married and has two children in primary school in Greenville. He is an active member of Southside Fellowship.

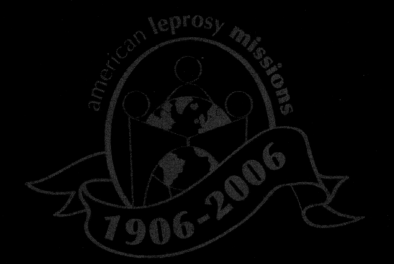

Part IV

Board of Directors

Giving direction to and providing continuity for this Mission during this centenary was a twenty- to thirty-member board. One hundred and thirty-nine dedicated persons have or are now serving in this capacity. Directors were without exception Christians, with membership in a variety of denominations, committed to ALM and its mission. They have given generously of their time without remuneration.

In the early years, the board was comprised entirely of men; in recent years, however, both genders have been well represented. Most directors served more than one three-year term; some served for most of a lifetime in either a field or a board capacity. Only two were themselves leprosy survivors. Prominent among them were physicians (thirty-eight), teachers, lawyers, businesspersons, ministers, and professors; a few qualified as scientists, and one was a former professional football player. Notable even in this elite circle was William Jay Schieffelin, who served the first forty years as chairman. All except three were Americans, although some served as overseas missionaries or executives.

Wherever possible, dates of service and city of residence are listed. If a date or city is not listed, that information is unavailable.

Justin E. Abbott, M.D.
1917

W. Espey Albig
Wassaic, N.Y. 1941–1953

Samuel A. Alward, vice chairman (1994–1997)
Washington, D.C. 1991–1999

Gerald H. Anderson
Ventnor, N.J. 1978–1982

Lloyd Auten
Greenville, S.C. 1966–1991

Dr. Wm. Ward Ayer
St. Petersburg, Fla. 1948–1962

Emily Bailey
Pauleys Island, S.C. 1999–present

Hugh Barfield
Wheaton, Ill. 1991–1999

Gerald F. Beavan
Phoenixville, Penn. 1979–1983

Dr. Reeve H. Betts
Drexel Hills, Penn. 1961–1970

W. E. Biederwolf, M.D.
Palm Beach, Fla. 1933

Rev. J. Blaine Blubaugh
Falls Church, Vir. 1990–1998

Margaret E. Brand, M.D.
Seattle, Wash. 1977–present

Harold N. Brewster, M.D.
New York, N.Y. 1960–1965

S. Edward Briggs
1921

Glen R. Brubaker, M.D.
Lancaster, Penn. 1997–present

Wolfe F. Bulle, M.D.
St. Louis, Mo. 1963–1979

John D. Burton, DD, chairman (1995–1997)
Richmond, Vir. 1988–1997

Howard S. Butterweck
Brookside, N.J. 1960–1971

Delmar R. Byler
Tenafly, N.J. 1983–1986

Don L. Calame
1964–1966

Naomi Carman
Greenbelt, Md. 1981–1989

Robert Carty
Lewisville, Tex. 1981–1989

Chamberlain, M.D.
1933

Carol Childs
Bethesda, Md. 1997–2004

Peter B. Christie
1955–1957

James D. Cockman, chairman (2001–2003)
Landrum, S.C. 1996–2004

Mrs. Wade Coggins
Kensington, Md. 1960

Douglas K. Comstock
Bevercreek, Ohio 1995–1997

Duvon C. Corbitt Jr., M.D.
New York, N.Y. 1972–1976

Douglas O. Corpron, M.D.
Yakima, Wash. 1987–1997

Caughey B. Culpepper
Atlanta, Ga. 1960–1963

Raymond Currier, honorary director
Croton-on-the-Hudson, N.Y. 1959–1970

Michael A. Cusick Jr., treasurer (1997–1999)
Venice, Fla. 1991–1999

John H. Dawson, M.D.
Mercer Island, Wash. 1987–present

Mrs. Robert DeLano
1961–1962

Paul M. Derstine
Hampstead, Md. 1999–2002

Larry E. Dixon
St. Simons Island, Ga. 1985–1994

Edward M. Dodd, M.D.
Montclair, N.J. 1948–1968

T. DeWitt Dodson
Westwood, N.J. 1960–1982

Addison J. Eastman
Lakewood, Ohio 1963–1982

Helen Erickson
Richfield, Minn. 1987–1992

M. J. Evans
Chicago, Ill. 1941–

Emanuel Faria
Carville, La. 1982–1994

Sheridan Farin
Chicago, Ill. 1948–1960

Harry Farmer
1923

James P. Fields, M.D.
Nashville, Tenn. 1978–present

Luther C. Fisher, III, M.D.
Houston, Tex. 1974–1977

Carroll B. Fitch
New York, N.Y. 1971–1977

Rev. Ernest L. Fogg, Th.D., chairman (1980–1984)
Montclair, N.J. 1978–1985

Rev. Gerald A. Foster, D.D., honorary director
Wilmington, Del. 1966–2000

Herbert H. Gass, M.D.
Pleasant Hill, Tenn. 1965–1977

Dr. Luther A. Gotwald
New York, N.Y. 1959–1963

Rev. Benjamin O. Gould, honorary director
Paoli, Penn. 2004

Edward D. Grant, honorary director (1981)
Baton Rouge, La. 1955–1980

E. P. Haggard, M.D.
New York, N.Y. 1917

Rev. F. B. Makepeace
1906

H. A. Manchester, D.D.
1909–1911

T. Grady Mangham Jr.
Nyack, N.Y. 1970–1977

Arnaud Marts, chairman (1959–1960)
Lewisburg, Penn. 1934–1963

Edward C. May
New York, N.Y. 1974–1980

William McColl, M.D., chairman (1988–1994)
La Jolla, Calif. 1968–2004

David McConaughy
Montclair, N.J. 1917

George W. McCoy, M.D.
1917

Donald McGilchrest
1983–1984

George F. McInnes
Augusta, Ga., 1961–1969

Pearl McNeil, Ph.D.
King of Prussia, Penn. 1979–1985

Wayne M. Meyers, M.D., Ph.D., chairman
(1984–1988)   Laurel, Md. 1979–2003

Timothy S. Midura, Esq.
Chicago, Ill. 1988–1996

Orie O. Miller, chairman (1960–1965); honorary
director (1974); Akron, Penn. 1958–1965

Mrs. Otis Moore
Garnersville, N.Y. 1947–1951

Minot Morgan, M.D.
1933

Wiley Henry Mosley
Baltimore, Md. 1987

Randall Nauman
1958–1961

J. Frederick Neudoerffer
New York, N.Y. 1960–1983

Bishop F. B. Newel
1958–1962

Frank D. Nicodem Sr.
Mount Prospect, Ill. 1972–1979

Mark Oleksak
Tampa, Fla. 2003–present

Julia Oliver
Jamesburg, N.J. 1985–1991

John D. Ordway
Greenwich, Conn. 1988–1991

Michael J. Pasnik
Basking Ridge, N.J. 1974–1976

S. J. Patterson Jr.
1958–1964

Helen E. Pedersen
Glenrock, N.J. 1972–1979

Ruben A. Pedersen, honorary director
Glenrock, N.J. 1958–1977

Rev. Dalavan L. Pierson
New York, N. Y. 1906–1937

Patricia Brand Peters
Mercer Island, Wash. 1996–2001

José Ramirez
Houston, Tex. 1999–present

Sandra Reiner
Chicago, Ill. 1991–2001

Dean Reule
Wesley Chapel, Fla. 1997–2002

Fleming H. Revell
New York, N. Y. 1906–1935

Dr. J. G. Vaughan
New York, N.Y. 1941–1947

Lorene Vychopen
Greenwich, Conn. 1977–1980

Mark H. Ward
Boston, Mass. 1948–1952

Margaret Weeks
New Orleans, La. 1959–1964

Rosa Page Welch
Denver, Colo. 1969–1979

Ruth Winant Wheeler
Buffalo, N.Y. 1971

Albert O. Wilson Jr.
Cambridge, Mass. 1960–1970

Mrs. James D. Wyker
1957–1961

Angus G. Wynne Jr., Esq.
Dallas, Tex. 1955–1961

Leo Yoder, M.D.
Baton Rouge, La. 1993–2001

Thomas M. Young
East Sandwich, Mass. 1980 –present

Executive Directors

Twelve men provided leadership during the first one hundred years of ALM. In the early years the title was general secretary, but in more recent years it was president, with the recent addition of CEO. In truth, they have all been executive directors. William Danner had the longest tenure with twenty-six years. Next in tenure were Oliver Hasselblad with fifteen years and Eugene Kellersberger with twelve years. A few served in an interim capacity. Most served previously in the mission field. It can be said that they "caught leprosy"! They served sacrificially, although they would not have said it that way.

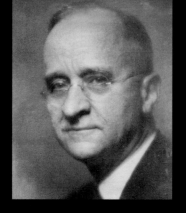

William Mason Danner
General Secretary, 1911–1937

William Mason Danner was the first full-time executive officer of the American Committee, which later became the American Mission to Lepers (AML), and in 1950 American Leprosy Missions (ALM). Appointed in 1911, Danner served as general secretary for twenty-six years. He had previously served with distinction as general secretary of the Young Men's Christian Association for more than twenty years while also working for the Kellogg Food Company.

Working out of an upstairs bedroom in his Cambridge, Massachusetts home, family and neighbors found themselves pressed into service assembling literature and stuffing envelopes. The office secretary lived with the Danner family. Mrs. Danner and their daughter, Lois, regularly attended meetings of the American Committee. They served without title and mostly without compensation. The office moved to Tremont Temple Church, Boston, in 1917. After being officially incorporated in New York on July 31, 1917, the office relocated to 156 Fifth Avenue, New York, where it remained until 1960.

During Danner's tenure, the American Mission to Lepers relied on the deputation of field secretaries and furloughing United States missionaries. Their messages heightened awareness of the plight of leprosy and the need for support first in India, but eventually also in Japan, China, Thailand, South America, and Africa. Danner traveled extensively organizing auxiliaries and raising awareness and support. In 1912 there were thirty-two auxiliaries and

councils in Canada and the USA. By 1914 the number jumped to sixty-three, eventually reaching approximately five hundred by 1930.

Danner's testimony before the U.S. Congress resulted in legislation that authorized the construction of a national leprosarium and instructed the surgeon general to prepare rules and regulations for patients to be admitted. Danner served on the committee that selected Carville, Louisiana, as the location for the first U.S.-based service with an objective of both treating leprosy and preventing its spread.

That accomplished, Danner directed his considerable energies to realizing a Protestant chapel at Carville, dedicated in 1924. Dr. George McCoy, long-time head of the National Institute of Health, wrote to Danner on the occasion of his retirement: "Not many people know it and fewer would say, but the splendid Federal Leprosarium at Carville is a monument to you and you alone."

An article in the *Star* stated simply: "If institutions are but the extended shadows of the men in whose mind they were conceived, then the shadow of one falls more definitely across Carville than does that of any other man. That man is William Mason Danner."

Danner was not a man inclined to settle into the narrow limits of his original tasks. By the time of his retirement in 1937, ALM was supporting programs in twenty-five countries in Europe, Africa, Asia, and both South and North America. Not only ALM's first executive officer, he has the distinction of having served longer in that capacity than any of his successors.

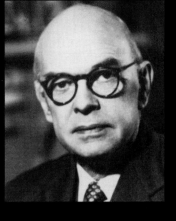

Emory Ross, M.D.
General Secretary, 1937–1941

Dr. Emory Ross came to ALM with a distinguished record of service in what was then Belgium Congo under the United Christian Missionary Society of the Disciples of Christ Church. Ross had also served as secretary of the Congo Christian Council, representing all Protestant missions in the Congo, and was widely known as an expert in African affairs.

Ross responded to ALM's call to become its second executive officer in 1937. He referred to himself as the "Stop-gap Secretary." He rendered four years of outstanding leadership before being elected to serve as vice chair for seven years, followed by eleven years as chairman—a total of twenty-four years.

Ross's legacy centered in fostering cooperation with mission groups and governments. Fundraising and promotional work had by this time been assigned to four established and functioning branch offices, each with its own field secretary and staff: New England in Boston; Midwest in Chicago; Pacific Coast in Los Angeles; and East Central in Atlanta.

Ross was instrumental in launching the special Five-Year Anti-Leprosy Postwar Fund campaign in 1944. It was through this fund that ALM became associated with the Vellore Christian Medical College and its pioneer, Dr. Ida B. Scudder.

Ross concluded his distinguished career in 1959.

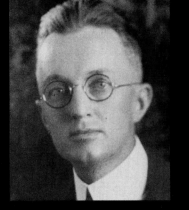

Eugene R. Kellersberger, M.D.
General Secretary, 1941–1953

Dr. Eugene R. Kellersberger took the helm as general secretary of American Mission to Lepers on March 15, 1941. Kellersberger was a recognized authority on tropical diseases that included sleeping sickness and leprosy. He founded and administered the leprosy colony sponsored by the Presbyterian Church (South) at Bibanga, Congo, and also served as secretary of the medical committee of the Congo Protestant Council. By appointment of King Leopold of Belgium, Kellersberger was a member of the Royal Commission for the protection of natives.

Recognizing his established abilities in fundraising and administration, and being in need of executive leadership, the AML board asked the Foreign Missions Committee of the Presbyterian Church to release Dr. Eugene and Mrs. Julia Lake Kellersberger for service as deputation speakers. This call came as the Kellersbergers were nearing twenty-five years of service in the Belgium Congo. Thus, in the spring of 1941, Kellersberger was appointed general secretary and his wife was appointed to serve as promotional secretary for the mission.

Soon after his appointment, Kellersberger increased the number of branch offices from four to six by adding offices in New Jersey and Texas. Additionally, four full-time field secretaries worked out of their homes.

One of his main emphases was building awareness for ALM initiatives both in the private and the governmental sectors, drawing heavily on his long experience in the Belgian Congo. This work eventually resulted in increased financial support to the mission.

During Kellersberger's tenure, ALM broadened its emphasis from custodial care to modern medical treatment, including prevention and rehabilitation; this involved special training for leprosy workers. The new emphasis led to heightened cooperation with the Ethiopian government, resulting in the establishment of a training program at the Princess Zenebework Hospital, later known as the All Africa Leprosy and Rehabilitation Training Centre (ALERT). It became the rallying point for growing leprosy programs on the African continent.

Under Kellersberger's leadership, a special medical fund was set up in 1947 to supply Promin and Dapsone drugs to "stations from which precise reports in the experimental use of these new drugs can be assured." In an effort to combat stigma associated with leprosy, he led the charge to change the name of the American Mission to Lepers to American Leprosy Missions. He presented a paper on stigma to a symposium of the New York Academy of Science in 1950. The emphasis on collaborating with missions and governments pioneered by Dr. Emory Ross was continued by Kellersberger and is part of his legacy.

In a search for ways to permanently honor the Kellersbergers upon their retirement in 1953, the Board of Directors elected him honorary vice president for life. Following Kellersberger's death, the Board of Directors entered into an agreement with ALERT, establishing (with ALM support) the annual Kellersberger Memorial Lecture, to be given by a "leprosy specialist of international renown."

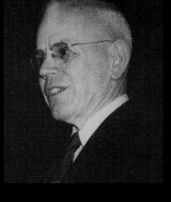

Following a prolonged search, Harold Hayes Henderson became general secretary of American Leprosy Missions in January 1954. A former missionary in Korea under the United Presbyterian Church, USA for twenty-one years, Henderson had served as principal of the Mission Boys' Academy and missionary pastor-evangelist for twenty churches.

The board instructed its new general secretary to enlarge the program and increase its support within the next five years, by which time was noted, he would reach standard retirement age. To achieve these goals, Henderson was authorized to hire a promotional secretary to supervise field representatives; augment the literature and publicity staff; and increase audio-visual capability including television, radio, film, and filmstrips.

In October 1954, the board approved exploring increased use of computers, resulting in the installation of Remington Rand equipment. Operations were transferred from the branch offices to the central headquarters, a decision that plagued ALM for many years.

To realize these ambitious educational and fund-raising goals, Henderson ventured into the use of new techniques. He made increased use of radio and explored the use of television, then in its infancy. Seven motion-picture films with descriptive brochures and nine color filmstrips with scripts were produced. In a four-month period, seventy-five televised bookings reached an estimated audience of 3,116,714 viewers. One station reported that they were "without a doubt the finest free films ever shown over WXNX."

In September 1955, *American Leprosy Missions News* was introduced as the new ALM organ. Henderson stated that, henceforth, publications, appeal letters, news, and information would originate in the New York headquarters rather than branch offices.

The golden jubilee anniversary of American Leprosy Missions was celebrated on October 17 and 18, 1956. The theme was "The Role of the Christian Church in the Fight Against Hansen's Disease (Leprosy)." Additionally, a series of conferences was conducted throughout the country.

Henderson resigned in June 1958, in a time of turmoil. It had fallen to him to lead the organization in a period of transition to greater centralization and the use of new technologies. It would be another fifteen years before the board was willing to consider a computerized approach to gifts and donor receipt processing.

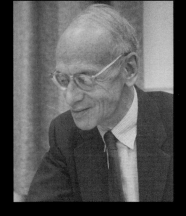

Raymond P. Currier
General Secretary, 1958–1960

Having served as executive secretary since 1936, Raymond P. Currier was elected to serve as general secretary in 1958 while the search continued for a permanent appointment. Currier's first association with ALM was in 1926 when he spent a summer working in the office while General Secretary William M. Danner toured overseas programs. Earlier he had taught in Burma under American Baptist Foreign Missions appointment. At various times he served on the ALM Finance Committee.

Currier was a poet-writer-administrator with an abiding interest in people and ideas. He raised money, made speeches, edited publications, produced literature, visited overseas treatment centers, administered both foreign and domestic programs, and above everything, loved and helped people everywhere. Ray Currier was clearly the go-to person in the years between 1930 and 1960; he possessed a natural approach to every problem.

While he served as executive secretary, the Board of Directors asked Currier to make an analysis of the Schramm Report related to money-raising procedures and effectiveness. Some believed overhead costs were too high. Currier concluded that the ALM cost of income generation was not excessive and that "an intensive effort toward the development of auxiliaries should yield large results and help reduce costs." The nature of voluntary auxiliaries was, Currier concluded, not well understood. "Work done through them is done at our expense. They are not self-supporting."

Ray Currier ended his long service with ALM in 1960. When Dr. Oliver Hasselblad was appointed, he requested that Currier be retained to help with the transition.

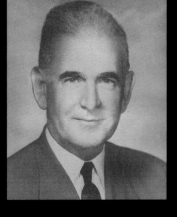

Edward D. Grant
Acting President, 1958–1959

Edward D. Grant declined an invitation to ascend to the presidency. Some months later he stated his willingness to accept a part-time, temporary appointment if the board felt this would be wise and beneficial to ALM. Grant became acting president, serving for one year. He remained associated with the board until his death on November 13, 1985.

Born in Glasgow, Scotland, Grant came to the United States at the age of twelve. He received his M.A. from Peabody Teachers College in Nashville, Tennessee. Two honorary degrees were conferred on him: Lit.D. from Austin College and LHD from Southwestern College in Memphis.

In 1921 Grant became secretary of education and promotion of the Foreign Board of the Presbyterian Church, U.S., in Nashville. From 1934 to 1952 he served as executive secretary of the Board of Christian Education. During this time he traveled widely. He was introduced to leprosy on a trip from 1929 to 1930 to the Far East.

Louisiana Governor R. P. Kennon appointed Grant to assume responsibility for the newly organized Board of Institutions in 1952, giving him authority over several dozen state institutions. For this work, Grant received the Distinguished Service Award from Louisiana College in 1954.

In his last report to the Board of Directors, Grant recommended strengthening relationships with mission boards and denominations related to the Division of Foreign Missions of the National Council of Churches, as well as the Evangelical Foreign Mission Association of the National Association of Evangelicals. Board size was increased to thirty, making room for executives from these boards to serve on the ALM Board of Directors.

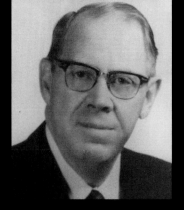

Oliver W. Hasselblad, M.D.
President, 1959–1974

D r. Oliver William Hasselblad became the seventh executive officer of ALM in 1959. A Baptist physician and surgeon, Hasselblad spent almost twenty years as a medical missionary in India. The British government awarded him the coveted Kaiser-I-Hind award for outstanding service. While medical director of the American Baptist Hospital at Jorhat, Assam, India, Hasselblad also supervised the Kangpokpi Leprosy Hospital in Manipur for three years. When Dr. and Mrs. Hasselblad took over the medical work at Jorhat, it was a small institution with twenty-five beds. When they left in 1957, it was a thriving community with a 225-bed general hospital including a TB ward, an enlarged leprosy settlement, and two out-lying medical units.

While at the University of Nebraska College of Medicine, Hasselblad pastored the Grace Baptist Church in Omaha. Upon graduation in 1936 he served two years of internship and surgical residency in St. Louis, Missouri, and Peru, Indiana. His graduate work included two years at Harvard and New York University and a year at the Cook County Post-Graduate School.

Hasselblad assumed the ALM presidency in a time of transition. Two board chairmen retired within eighteen months and the number of field representatives was reduced from eight veterans to six new recruits. There was also the challenge of implementing a complex reorganization plan.

The Board of Directors added to the load by instructing its new president to review the support arrangement of the India program. This called into question the long-standing cooperative arrangement, indeed, the parent-child relationship that had prevailed for more than fifty years.

In January 1960, in an effort to bring expenses in line with income, Hasselblad recommended reducing the number of regional offices to four and expanding the office of president by absorbing the duties formerly performed by the general secretary and director of field program.

A further challenge emerged when, in 1960, the building that had long housed ALM at 156 Fifth Avenue, New York City was sold, causing ALM to relocate to 297 Park Avenue South. The expanded and improved facilities were welcome; the added expense was not.

Hasselblad inherited four key staff members including Ms. Helen Rozenweig, staff secretary since Mr. Danner's time. In due course he added Dr. Glen W. Tuttle, administrative vice president; Eugene L. Wilson, controller; John R. Sams, administrative vice president; and Robert M. Bradburn, director of development. With the exception of Tuttle's 1972 retirement, this team served through the late 1980s, with Eugene Wilson serving into the new millennium.

At Hasselblad's urging, the board adopted comprehensive policy statements encompassing Christian witness, prevention, control, treatment, rehabilitation, and programs to support patients returning to community life.

ALM raised over $1.385 million in 1959, the highest in its history, supporting a staff of twenty-four workers. Hasselblad had extraordinary ability to attract and challenge talented staff. He traveled extensively for evaluation and information gathering purposes, visiting every

ALM-supported hospital, clinic, or leprosy program, even in remote villages. He made nearly forty overseas trips, some of six weeks' duration.

Dr. Oliver William Hasselblad retired from ALM on June 1, 1974, but continued as medical consultant until 1975. He then assisted the Government of Jamaica in devising a leprosy control program and later served as medical administrator for Kalaupapa Settlement on the island of Molokai, Hawaii.

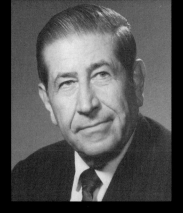

Roger K. Ackley
President, 1974–1981

The election of Rev. Roger K. Ackley represented a new beginning for ALM. Ackley began his varied career as a youth worker in California. During World War II he elected to work with Japanese families held in prison-like internment camps. In the post-war era Ackley was appointed to the staff of USAID Egypt, remaining in that Muslim nation for ten years. Thereafter, he served with the United Nations High Commission for Refugees with assignments in Europe and in Vietnam. Finally and briefly, he worked for KLM Royal Dutch Airlines, helping it to secure landing rights in Chicago. This qualified him to travel extensively at little or no cost to ALM.

Soon after his appointment, Ackley convinced the board to move the headquarters from its location in New York City to a small suburban community in Bloomfield, New Jersey. This resulted in savings in personnel and administrative costs. He invited Dr. W. Felton Ross, director of training at ALERT, and Dr. Roy Pfaltzgraff, a missionary returning home from Nigeria, to join the ALM headquarters staff. Following the board's directive to emphasize financial growth through church-based and general public education programs, Ackley promoted the World Leprosy Day. He also worked with interchurch agencies and reached out to denominational leaders, chaplains, and pastors. For the first time since ALM's disastrous early experience with computers in the mid 1950s, Ackley convinced the board to computerize the ALM mailing list.

The European Federation of Anti-Leprosy Associations (ELEP) had by this time changed its name from the European Federation to the International Federation of Anti-Leprosy Associations (ILEP), permitting ALM to join. Membership in this International consortium of leprosy organizations allowed ALM to expand its work to more than thirty countries and facilitated integrated programs with governmental health ministries.

ILEP also promoted the development of regional training and research centers including those at Karigiri, India; ALERT in Ethiopia; and the Institute Lauro de Souza Lima (ISLI) in Brazil. Research was emphasized, as field reports indicated that patients were becoming resistant to dapsone treatment. Unbeknown to this generation of dedicated leprosy workers, a research breakthrough was in the making.

Roger Ackley's tenure with ALM ended with his retirement on August 31, 1981.

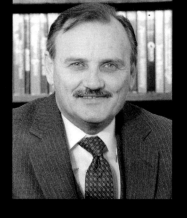

Dr. Waldron "Scottie" Scott was elected to a five-year term as president of ALM in May 1981. Formerly with The Navigators, and general secretary of the World Evangelical Fellowship, Scott was a frequent contributor to religious periodicals. He won acclaim by a brilliantly written book, *Bring Forth Justice*, stressing the integral relationship between mission, discipleship, and social justice—three values high on the ALM search committee's list.

Scott left immediately after his appointment to survey ALM partner agencies and programs on a world tour. The trip's purpose, he said, was to strengthen ALM relationships with the Leprosy Mission (London) and the Philippine Leprosy Mission. The World Health Organization had just reported success with the use of multiple drugs in treating leprosy on the Island of Malta. "Leprosy can now be cured and perhaps eliminated," Scott proclaimed boldly to a skeptical board.

The board approved his recommendation to use the name "ALM International" instead of "American Leprosy Missions," de-emphasizing the word leprosy. A working group on leprosy and social justice reviewed new opportunities and directions for Christian health-care ministries working towards the year 2000. The board shared, with some enthusiasm, Scott's May 1983 report labeled "Shifting into High Gear," calling on ALM to join in the effort to eradicate Hansen's disease by the year 2000.

John R. Sams, executive vice president, and Robert M. Bradburn, director of development, had visions for using television as a fund-raising medium. The board approved Scott's recommendation to proceed with the production of television as a major fund-raising tool. At the May 1982 board meeting, Scott unveiled an aggressive five-year-plan calling for major expansion in overseas programs and the United States support base. Scott's big dream featured new forms of therapy; it removed barriers to integrated care; and concentrated on caring for people with disabilities. The office staff increased from eighteen to twenty-eight in 1982, and resources were expected to come from television income, which was projected to reach fifteen million dollars annually.

ALM's first television special, "Don't Let it Happen to the Children," showed great promise. Mail volume was five times greater than in the previous year. The office staff and new computer were hard-pressed to keep up with the almost tripling of new donors and contributions. Scott projected that contributions would rise to $3.3 million by year's end, a 37.5 percent increase over the previous year.

Amid this frenzy, the board of directors was mystified to learn that field remittances needed to fulfill the five-year-plan were in arrears. Overhead expenses were up sharply due to increased staff and a new office complex located across the river in Bloomfield, New Jersey. The treasurer reported to a stunned board that field commitments of more than $500,000 would be carried over into 1984.

Waldron Scott resigned the presidency in July 1984; it was a short but exhilarating period in ALM's history.

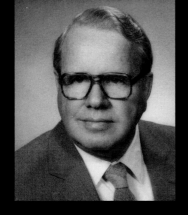

John R. Sams
President, 1984–1989

everend John R. Sams was confirmed as ALM's tenth executive officer in November 1984. Sams was born and received his education in Iowa before attending Hartford Theological School in Connecticut. Following forty-two months in the U.S. Air Force, he obtained his master's degree in counseling from Chapman College in Orange, California. Sams spent seventeen years as a missionary under the Christian Church (Disciples of Christ), serving in the Philippines, where he was director of the United Missionary office, coordinating the work of six Protestant church denominations.

Sams joined the ALM staff in 1972 as administrative vice president. In 1982, he attended the Columbia University Institute for Not-For-Profit Management. Having served as executive vice president and program director under two presidents, and having traveled widely in Asia, he was well prepared for the difficult role that faced him when he was asked to serve as ALM's acting president in 1984. Field remittances were in arrears and ways needed to be found to promote the ALM program in an increasingly competitive environment.

Sams was also acquainted with ILEP, having been in attendance in Venice in 1984 when the World Health Organization (WHO) recommended multidrug therapy (MDT) as the treatment of choice. The availability of the long-awaited cure called for dramatic program shifts, requiring closer cooperation with governments and national voluntary agencies. Several pilot treatment programs were established to accelerate adoption of this new drug therapy. The ALM board was convinced to adopt the WHO recommendation when, in an experiment of less than three months, seventy-nine of one hundred patients were declared clinically cured of leprosy.

Under Sams's direction, staffing was reconfigured to respond to these program changes and to bring expenses in line with income. With reluctant board approval, he launched cautiously into the world of television acquisition. This proved to be at least a qualified success, helping ALM restore its strength and financial stability.

Although actively involved in the administration of field programs, Sams also freed himself to represent ALM at churches, conferences, and ILEP meetings. He maintained an active list of major donors whose contributions he personally acknowledged by telephone. He was instrumental in securing the first USAID grant for training programs in Guyana and during his tenure, the ALM budget grew from less than three million to more than nine million dollars. Sams attended ILEP meetings regularly and served on its executive committee for several years.

Sams retired from ALM in 1989. His years were among ALM's best in service and growth. The Christian University of the Philippines conferred on him an honorary doctor of humanities degree with a citation recognizing his contribution as a member of the National Leprosy Advisory Board of the Philippines.

Thomas Ferran Frist became president of ALM in 1989, bringing with him extensive international and field experience. A graduate of Davidson College, Frist also studied in France and Spain, and taught English literature in India on a Fulbright grant. He served as a UNICEF field representative in Vietnam, performed leprosy research in Tanzania with grants from Yale University, and studied Venezuela's leprosy programs.

Frist's career with ALM began in 1973 by being seconded to CERPHA Brazil. His assignment was to develop programs for communities of ex-leprosy patients who had been discharged from institutions but rejected by society. Working with Jorge de Macedo, executive director of CERPHA, and with directors of what became the Instituto Lauro de Souza Lima, they developed a pilot project, PRO-REHAB. It revamped how people affected by leprosy were treated in hospitals and health centers.

In 1976, Frist founded and directed SORRI ("smile" in Portuguese) in Bauru, Brazil. The first vocational rehabilitation program of its kind, it served all types of disabled persons, helping to train them vocationally, and integrating them into society. SORRI centers were eventually established in five Brazilian cities. Frist also helped found MORHAN, a national organization run primarily by persons affected by leprosy. It lobbies the Brazilian government in matters related to the treatment of leprosy.

During his almost-five years as ALM's president, Frist was instrumental in relocating the headquarters from Elmwood Park, New Jersey, to Greenville, South Carolina. He worked to broaden ALM's mission, giving more emphasis to people disabled by causes other than leprosy. Concerned about the stigma attached to segregated and sometimes paternalistic treatment programs, and by use of the word "leprosy," Frist emphasized integrated programs with patient participation.

Combating stigma was another strong theme of his administration. He supported the campaign to use the term Hansen's disease instead of leprosy.

Under Frist's leadership, ALM helped host the fourteenth International Leprosy Congress in 1993 in Orlando, Florida, the first such congress to be held in the United States. In 1994 Frist was elected to serve as president of the International Federation of Anti-Leprosy Agencies (ILEP), the only ALM person to serve in this capacity. He also served as chairman of the ILEP Working Group on the Social Aspects of Anti-Leprosy Work.

After leaving ALM in 1994, Frist continued as an advocate for leprosy-affected people. His book, *Don't Treat Me Like I Have Leprosy*, is used by many field projects around the world. He has published articles on Hansen's disease and rehabilitation in scientific journals, and has written a novel about leprosy called *The Descendant*. Frist served as a consultant to the Pan American Health Organization (PAHO) and on committees of the World Health Organization.

Christopher J. Doyle became the twelfth president and chief executive officer of ALM in January 1995. After a brief career in the U.S. Marine Corps, he graduated cum laude from Columbia International University in Columbia, South Carolina. Before coming to ALM in 1995, Doyle was the South Carolina state director of Bethany Christian Services.

In this multidrug-therapy era with shrinking leprosy registers, Doyle has retained the ALM commitment to leprosy while expanding the focus to what is becoming known as leprosy plus. This includes care after cure and also addresses other debilitating and stigmatizing diseases.

The overseas field staff has been expanded, coordinators have been appointed in major countries, and regional specialists have been added.

ALM now has field offices in Angola, D.R. Congo, Brazil, Myanmar, India, and the Philippines, plus two regional specialists in Prevention of Disability (POD) serving Asia, Africa, and South America. More emphasis is being given to "Cure Plus" including community-based rehabilitation projects, housing projects, basic education for children, and prevention of disability.

In 2001 ALM expanded its focus to include Buruli ulcer, an equally tragic and debilitating skin disease caused by an organism closely related to leprosy. It is prevalent in the West African countries of Ghana, Cote d'Ivoire, and Democratic Republic of the Congo.

ALM reduced the number of countries where it has active programs from twenty-seven to fifteen countries, permitting concentration on those where leprosy continues to be a major health problem. This has brought about increased focus and permits ALM to direct its efforts where it can be most effective.

An enthusiastic fundraiser, Doyle has brought innovation and persistence to this never-ending task. After many years of decline in numbers, ALM's donor base has grown by more than 10 percent to thirty-three thousand active donors. Starting in 1999, ALM began to receive funding from USAID through the American Schools and Hospitals Abroad (ASHA) program for Karigiri in India. To date, over $500,000 has been received from ASHA. Doyle has also expanded ALM's major donor program and foundation grants. In 2002, ALM's program budget hit an all-time high of $5.3 million. ALM has a goal of having fifty thousand active donors by 2008, and doubling its budget by 2014.

As part of its vision to "free the world of leprosy," under Doyle's leadership, ALM has undertaken its first $6.9-million capital campaign for vaccine research.

Doyle has served on the ILEP standing committee and several action groups, and served on the boards of the Schieffelin Leprosy Research & Training Center in Karigiri, India, and the Leprosy Mission Trust, India. In an effort to form closer ties between ALM and its founding parent, TLMI, Doyle has also served on its National Directors' Forum. He has traveled extensively, visiting ALM projects around the world and sharing his faith, vision, and commitment with field partners and with people affected by leprosy.

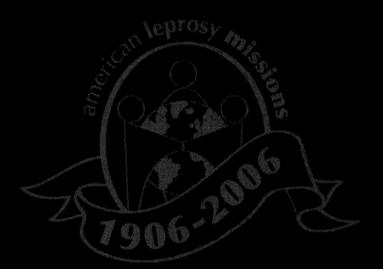

Appendices

Appendix A
ALM EXPENDITURES BY YEAR compiled by Eugene Wilson

1906–1925		1926–1945		1946–1965		1966–1985		1986–2006	
1906	$6,122	1926	$118,545	1946	$579,788	1966	$775,959	1986	$7,117,231
1907	$4,078	1927	$145,245	1947	$601,062	1967	$850,660	1987	$8,328,896
1908	$4,466	1928	$202,780	1948	$647,225	1968	$675,842	1988	$8,051,467
1909	$11,602	1929	$220,043	1949	$627,909	1969	$950,042	1989	$7,189,937
1910	$14,598	1930	$254,692	1950	$715,527	1970	$981,231	1990	$7,972,892
1911	$22,758	1931	$147,666	1951	$685,445	1971	$952,324	1991	$7,102,287
1912	$19,069	1932	$113,915	1952	$813,252	1972	$971,162	1992	$7,258,749
1913	$28,090	1933	$107,837	1953	$810,590	1973	$1,265,089	1993	$6,557,869
1914	$28,143	1934	$110,928	1954	$748,701	1974	$1,250,481	1994	$4,996,543
1915	$34,269	1935	$134,497	1955	$783,870	1971	$1,133,967	1995	$5,143,205
1916	$38,347	1936	$165,621	1956	$849,258	1976	$1,141,656	1996	$5,356,352
1917	$42,813	1937	$186,751	1957	$816,153	1977	$1,223,368	1997	$6,378,162
1918	$54,415	1938	$186,070	1958	$823,451	1978	$1,427,998	1998	$6,242,292
1919	$60,013	1939	$199,092	1959	$764,729	1979	$1,460,475	1999	$6,985,552
1920	$65,135	1940	$214,179	1960	$715,013	1980	$1,619,920	2000	$7,134,932
1921	$71,213	1941	$246,112	1961	$788,582	1981	$2,085,939	2001	$7,702,994
1922	$83,291	1942	$298,839	1962	$781,650	1982	$2,192,819	2002	$8,149,003
1923	$88,835	1943	$403,939	1963	$547,906	1983	$3,576,861	2003	$7,711,977
1924	$91,437	1944	$499,372	1964	$783,289	1984	$3,797,377	2004	$7,126,960
1925	$97,035	1945	$572,124	1965	$808,969	1985	$4,539,079	2005	$7,333,000

TOTALS

	$865,729		$4,528,247		$14,692,369		$32,872,249		$139,840,300

TOTAL: $192,798,894

Author's Note: In comparison, in A Journey of Mercy, *Oliver Hasselblad reported that receipts from 1897 through 1927 (thirty years) totaled $1,444,952.22; and from 1928 through 1934 (seven years) totaled $1,284,563.77.*

227

Appendix B

ALM PARTNERS compiled by Eugene Wilson

Through the years, American Leprosy Missions has collaborated with a wide variety of organizations including mission societies, national churches, agencies, and governments. Two hundred and thirty are listed here. We apologize for any that may have been missed.

ADRA International—Adventist Church
Africa Evangelical Fellowship
Africa Inland Mission
African Methodist Episcopal Church
Alfredo de Mato Dermatologic Center, Manaus, Brazil
Alliance Missionaire Évangélique
All Africa Leprosy, Tuberculosis and Rehabilitation Training Centre (ALERT), Ethiopia
Amazon Basin Benevolent Association (ABBA)
American Baptist Churches
American Council of Voluntary Agencies for Foreign Service, Inc.
American Schools and Hospitals Abroad (ASHA)
American Methodist Episcopal Mission
American Leprosy Foundation (Leonard Wood Memorial)
American Registry of Pathology
AMEXTRA, Puebla, Mexico
Amity Foundation, The
Aramboly Vocational Training Centre, India
Assistência Evangélica aos Doentes de Lepra, Portugal
Asociación Evangélica Mennonita del Paraguay
Association for Helping the Hopeless
Association Française Raoul Follereau
Association of Evangelical Relief and Development Organization (AERDO)
Associazione Italiana Amici di Raoul Follereau
Beulah Land Services
BMMF/INTER SERVE
British Leprosy Relief Association
Cameroun Baptist Missions
Canadian Leprosy Council
Canadian Presbyterian Mission
Cardinal Leger Institute Against Leprosy, Canada
Chikballapur Hospital, India
Chinese Mission to Lepers
Chit Aree School (Lampang Leprosy Foundation), Thailand
Christian Blind Mission International, Inc.

Christian & Missionary Alliance
Christian Missions in Many Lands
Christian Fellowship Community Health Centre, Ambilikkai, India
Christian Fellowship Society, India
Christian Medical Association of India
Christian Medical Board of Tanzania
Christian Medical Commission of the World Council of Churches
Christian Reformed Church
Christu-Kula Ashram & Hospital, India
Church of Christ in Thailand
Church of Christ in Zaire
Church of South India
Church of the Brethren
Church World Service and Witness
Citrolandia Public Health Clinic, Brazil
Colonia di Marituba Rehabilitation Center, Belem, Brazil
Comite Executif de L'ordre de Malte Pour L'assistance Aux Lépreux (CIOMAL)
CODEL (Coordination in Development)
Comissão Evangélica de Reabilitação de Pacientes de Hanseníase, (CERPHA) Brazil
Communauté Évangelique au Centre de l'Afrique
Comprehensive Rural Health Project, Jamkhed, India
Conselho das Igrejas Evangélicas de Angola Central
Council of Baptist Churches in North East India
Curitiba Rehabilitation Program, Brazil
Damien-Dutton Society
Damien Foundation Belgium
Danish Mission Board of the Moravian Church
Daughters of Charity of St. Vincent de Paul
Department of Health, Philippines
Department of Health & Human Services, National Hansen's Disease Program, USA
Disciples of Christ
Diocese of Livingstone, The Catholic Church, Zambia

Duque de Caxias Health Center, Brazil
Eastern Mennonite Board of Missions & Charities
Eastern Mennonite Missions
Eastern Shan State Leprosy Mission
Eglise Evangélique Des Amis Du Burundi
Eglise Presbyterienne Camerounaise
Ellen Thoburn Cowen Memorial Hospital , Kolar, India
Episcopal Church, The
Equip Inc.
Evangelical Covenant Church
Evangelical Foreign Missions Association (EFMA) or Evangelical Fellowship of Mission Agencies
Evangelical Free Church of America
Evangelical Presbyterian Church of Ghana
FEBA Radio
Federal University of Rio de Janeiro, Brazil
FJKM Madagascar
Fondation Luxembourgeoise Raoul Follereau, Luxembourg
Gemeinde Komitee, Paraguay
German Leprosy Relief Association
Global Health Council (formerly National Council of International Health)
Global Outreach Missions
Goodwill Industries of America, Inc.
Government of Korea
Habitat for Humanity International
HANDA Rehabilitation and Welfare Association
Hansenologia Internationalis
Hatigar Leprosarium, India
Heifer Project International
Hind Kusht Nivaran Sangh, India
Hope Haven, Inc.
Hoskote Mission Hospital Center, India
Hospital São Francisco de Asís, Bambuí, Brazil
Igreja Episcopal do Brasil Diocese Central
Indian Association of Leprologists
Institut Lauro de Souza Lima, São Paulo, Brazil
Institut Medical Chretien du Kasai, Zaire
Institut Medical Evangélique, Zaire
International Association for Integration, Dignity and Economic Advancement (IDEA)
International Center for Training and Research in Leprosy and Related Diseases, Venezuela
International Federation of Anti-Leprosy Associations (ILEP)
International Leprosy Association

International Leprosy Union
International Nepal Fellowship
Jilib Primary Health Care Program, Somalia
Joni & Friends
Jorhat Christian Medical Center
Karanjpada Clinic, India
Kentung Leprosy Program, Myanmar
KOZENSHA, Japan
Lampang Leprosy Foundation, Thailand
Leonard Wood Memorial Research Center, Philippines
Lesa de Andrade Public Health Center, Recife, Brazil
Leprosy Trust Board, New Zealand
Leprosy Relief Work, Emmaus-Switzerland
Le Secours aux Lépreux, Canada
Lutheran Church in America
Lutheran Coordination Service of Tanzania
McKean Rehabilitation Institute, Thailand
Manoram Christian Hospital, Thailand
MAP International
Marathi Missions, India
Mar Thoma Church, India
Medical Ambassadors International
Medical Centers of West Africa
Mennonite Central Committee
Ministry of Health, Angola
Ministry of Health, Brazil
Ministry of Health, Chhattisgarh, India
Ministry of Health, Democratic Republic of the Congo
Ministry of Health, Ethiopia
Ministry of Health, Ghana
Ministry of Health, Guizhou Province, China
Ministry of Health, Ivory Coast, Côte d'Ivoire
Ministry of Health, Mexico
Ministry of Health, Myanmar
Ministry of Health, Perú
Ministry of Health, Rio de Janeiro State, Brazil
Ministry of Health, São Paulo State, Brazil
Misão Evangélica Filafricana, Angola
Mission Aviation Fellowship
Moravian Church in Western Tanzania
Moulmein Christian Leprosy Hospital, Myanmar
Myanmar Christian Leprosy Mission
National Association of Evangelicals (USA)
National Council of Churches of Christ

in the USA
National Institute for Medical Research
Nekursini Hospital, India
Nepal Leprosy Trust
Netherlands Leprosy Relief
North American Baptist Conference
North American Baptist General Missionary
    Society
Nova Iquacu Health Center, Brazil
Oasis—ABIAH Brazil
Oswaldo Cruz Institute, Brazil
Overseas Missionary Fellowship
Padre Bento Hospital, Brazil
Palavra & Ação, Brazil
Pan American Health Organization (PAHO)
Philippine Leprosy Mission
Presbyterian Church of Cameroun
Presbyterian Church in the United States
President's Committee on the Employment of the
    Handicapped
Prison Fellowship India
Project Grace, China
Rädda Barnen, Sweden
Reformed Church in America
Rehabilitation International, USA
Red Barnet, Denmark
Redd Barna, Norway
Roman Catholic Church, Divine World Order
Roman Catholic Church, Ethiopian Catholic
    Secretariat
Sanatorio San Francisco de Borja, Spain
Sasakawa Memorial Health Foundation, Japan
São Gonçalo Public Health Center, Brazil
Schieffelin Leprosy Research & Training Centre,
    Karigiri, India
Serving Humanity in Crisis (SHIC)
Sir J. J. Group of Hospitals, Bombay, India
Society of the Immaculate Heart of Mary, India
Solidariedade Evangélica (SOLE)
Sociedade Para a Rehabilitacão e Reintegracão do
    Incapacitado (SORRI), Brazil
Soure Missionarie della Consolata, Italy
Southern Presbyterian Church, US
Sudan Interior Mission (SIM USA)
Sudan United Mission, England
Sudan United Mission, South Africa

Swiss Alliance Mission
Tabriz Mission, Persia (Iran)
Taiwan Leprosy Relief Association
Tamil Nadu Voluntary Health Training Program,
    India
Tansen Hospital, Nepal
Tanzania Mennonite Church
T.E.A.M.—Nepal
THELEP, Belgium
The Leprosy Mission International
The Leprosy Mission Trust India
The Philippine Leprosy Coordinating Council
Trans World Radio
The Salvation Army, Catherine Booth Hospital,
    Aramboly, India
Trinidad Tobago Leprosy Relief Association
United Church Board of for World Ministries
United Church of Canada
United Church of Christ in the USA
United Lutheran Mission, Virgin Islands,
    West Indies
United Methodist Church in Central Zaire
United Methodist Church in Mozambique
United Methodist Church in Southern Asia
United Methodist Church of Liberia
United Methodist Church, USA
United Methodist Committee on Relief (UMCOR)
United Mission to Nepal
United Presbyterian Church in the USA
United States Public Health Service,
    Carville, Louisiana
University of Hawaii, School of Medicine
Vadala Leprosy Control Center
Vellore Christian Medical College & Hospital
Vellore Christian Medical College Board
Wilson Leprosy Center, Soonchun, Korea
WLEREC Protective Footwear Project, The
    Netherlands
Women's Foreign Missionary Society, Methodist
    Episcopal Church
World Concern
World Evangelical Fellowship
World Health Organization (WHO)
World Missions Far Corners
World Vision International

Appendix C

ALM AROUND THE WORLD compiled by Eugene Wilson

Following is a list of sixty-five countries where ALM has had program participation:

AFRICA
Angola
Benin
Burundi
Cameroon
Cape Verde
Central Africa Republic
Comoro Islands
Congo
Democratic Republic of Congo (Zaire)
Ethiopia
Ghana
Guinea Bissau
Ivory Coast (Côte d'Ivoire)
Kenya
Liberia
Madagascar
Malawi
Mali
Mozambique
Papua New Guinea
Niger
Nigeria
Rwanda
Somalia
South Africa
Tanzania
Uganda
Zambia

ASIA
Bangladesh
China
India
Indonesia
Japan
Korea
Myanmar (Burma)
Nepal
Pakistan
Philippines
Singapore
Taiwan (Formosa)
Thailand
Vietnam

SOUTH AMERICA
Brazil
Chile
Colombia
Guyana
Paraguay
Perú
Suriname
Venezuela

MEXICO, CENTRAL AMERICA, and the CARIBBEAN
Costa Rica
Cuba
Jamaica
México
Nicaragua
Panama
Trinidad and Tobago

EUROPE
Belgium
France
Great Britain
Netherlands
Portugal

MIDDLE EAST
Egypt
Persia (Iran)

UNITED STATES (Including)
Hawaii
Louisiana
Puerto Rico
Virgin Islands

231

Appendix D

"TOUCH"

by Paul W. Brand, C.B.E., M.B., B.S., F.R.C.S.

Chairman, Medical Consultative Committee

Address Delivered to Annual Meeting of American Leprosy Missions, Inc.

October 17, 1963

I believe that if we are to exist with any worthwhile purpose in our lives, it is to follow in the steps of our Master and to seek to do in some way what He did, and what He still wants to do through us. And I would like to base my thoughts on an action of our Lord, Jesus Christ, which was repeated over and over and over again, probably every day of His public ministry. Jesus reached out His hand and touched the man who was sick, the woman who was faint, and the people who needed Him.

I have sometimes wondered why Jesus Christ touched the people whom He healed. He could so easily, with that same power, have waved a magic wand. In fact, a wand would have reached more people than a touch. But we don't hear at any time that our Lord Jesus went about attacking diseases in that way. No, His mission was to people, to individual people, people who might happen to have a disease. They might come to Him because they had a disease, but He touched them because they were people, because they were human and because He loved them, and because in the healing act our Lord, Jesus Christ, wanted those people to feel His love, warmth, His identification with them, one by one.

You can't really demonstrate love to a crowd. If we really want to express love, it's hand to hand. As you grasp a hand, as you hold it, you are communicating something of yourself, something of your strength and your courage and your faith and your love.

And so I love the thought of touch. To me it is a miracle. And I think perhaps the reason that touch means most to me is that the people I work with, the patients whom I try to serve in India, practically all of them, have completely lost from their hands and their feet the feeling of touch. They put their hand on wood, they put it on metal, they put it on a soft fabric like velvet or the cold dewy grass in the morning and they all feel the same. There is no touch at all. And they put their hands on a hot, burning stove and it feels just the same as cool grass, and their hands get burned and their hands get destroyed, and very few people can survive a lifetime without touch without destroying most of their fingers and perhaps both of their feet.

And so, as I see these dear people who have so much to bear, slowly and gradually and little by little, losing the fingers which should be the instruments of their capacity to earn their living, through which they should receive the warmth of human fellowship, as I see those fingers twisted and gnarled and insensitive, I hate leprosy. And the thing that I hate about it more than any other thing is that it destroys touch. It takes away the sensation of pain, it cuts me off from my fellow men because they can't feel me when I hold their hands.

And you know the person with leprosy loses touch in more than one way. Not only does this horrible disease get into the nerves of his arms and destroy them and strangle them so that he can never again feel with his fingers, but somehow, and for some reason that I cannot understand, this same germ gets between him and his friends, gets between him and his employer, gets between him and his community and builds a barrier, so that a man who had experienced the loving, warm greetings of his friends before, who had a job and could earn his living, finds that people turn away, that the children will run from him because they have been told by their parents that they mustn't associate with this man who has leprosy. He is treated with a superstitious kind of fear. And so it is that leprosy is a lonely disease. Leprosy is a lonely disease!

My wife could tell you of the loneliest people of all. They are the ones for whom leprosy has also destroyed their sight. And so, like many another in the world, they are blinded, but unlike most of the blind they can't use their hands to bring them the sensations that their eyes are denied because they can't feel either. They are really alone.

Sometimes I am asked, "Why do you need a leprosy mission? Leprosy surely is a disease. Leprosy is caused by a germ. You don't have a mission for chicken pox or a mission for various infectious diseases. They are treated by public health organizations—they are treated by government medical officers. Why does a Christian church need to get into this business of treating leprosy in such a special way? Why single out this one disease?"

The answer to that question lies in what we have just been saying—because more than any other person in the world the person with leprosy needs to be treated by somebody who will reach out his hand in the name of the Lord Jesus and touch him because, in that personal touch backed by love and affection and devotion and compassion, we are mediating the love of Jesus Christ that this man, isolated by the world, should be welcomed into the fellowship of the Lord Jesus Christ.

Many a time, when working with a leprosy patient to restore paralyzed hands, to build up a deformed foot, and I have been able to restore him to something which is acceptable to society, I think that the thing that he appreciated most in the whole process of scientific rehabilitation and reconstruction is that when he first came into our fellowship we reached out and we took his hand in our hands and we loved him. Oh, I have

seen men break down into tears at that time because they have found someone who would touch them. And this is the authentic mission of the Church.

I want to tell you the story of a leprosy patient who came to me through a remarkable woman, my mother, because this story demonstrates all three aspects of what ALM, as a mission, is trying to do. The patient I'm thinking about was a beggar. He had had leprosy for years, ever since he had been a little child, and he wandered around the villages in a mountain range where there were no schools, no shops, no post offices, no roads— nothing—just a wild mountain range. This boy went from village to village begging his food. He didn't have a complete finger on either hand. Each of his fingers was a little bit damaged or partly destroyed. Both of his feet were partly worn away with constant and chronic ulcerations. He was a miserable specimen of humanity, but there was somebody who loved miserable specimens of humanity, and that was my old mother.

She became a missionary in south India, in the hills, when she was a young woman. At age 65 she was told to retire because the mission couldn't keep people after 65. And so she retired, but she found a new range of mountains where there never was a missionary. She climbed those mountains all by herself and built a little wooden shack on the top, and there she worked for 20 years. She was nearly 80 when this boy came there. She had broken one leg and couldn't walk except with two sticks, but she had a noble horse, and on the back of this horse she rode all over the mountains, with a little medical box behind her on the saddle, to seek out the unwanted and the unlovely and the sick and the halt and the maimed and the blind and bring treatment to them. She recognized this young beggar boy's leprosy and felt that his troubles were a little beyond what she could do. So she came down to the foot of the hills with him on her horse, got him to the third class compartment of a rattly old train, and she came with him to our hospital, a hundred miles away, and she handed him over to me.

And we saw these feet, grossly deformed and ulcerated, and these hands, twisted and distorted, and there didn't seem very much hope for a boy like that. But we took him in. I suppose I was bullied by my mother. We knew it was going to take a long time because both of his hands and every one of his fingers needed operations, and both of his feet needed to be healed. He had to be a bed patient and have all attention. I believe it was a full year before we discharged that boy, after a number of operations. He hadn't any leprosy by that time, in any case, and his fingers were working again and he seemed very happy.

At that same time, we had been doing some research work trying to find out the kind of shoes that would prevent trophic ulcerations of the feet in leprosy, that would protect these feet that were so liable to injury as they walked over rough ground. As a parting gift, we presented the boy with a pair of these lovely shoes, some of the first experimental models that we had made of the shoes that proved so successful later on.

And all the time he was in that hospital, cared for by the nurses, by the paramedical workers, by the doctors, something else had happened. Some of his fellow patients had talked with him, and some of those who were literate had taught him to read, and he had been reading his Bible. He realized that a whole new world was opening up before him. He had come into a community of people who loved the Lord God, and who were keen that he should go back as a MAN, with dignity. When he went back to the hills, to my old mother, he told her he wanted to follow the Lord, Jesus Christ, and to become the first, the foundation member of the church up in those hills.

I went to visit a little while later. He was now working. He had become a teacher. They say that in the country of the blind, the one-eyed man is king. In a mountain range where nobody can read, the man who can say "a, b, c's" is a teacher, and so he had a little school going, the children from all around coming to him. He was beginning to be a person who was looked up to and respected, and he was doing a little farming.

But one thing was very tragic. As I looked at his feet there were the old bandages around them again. I said to him, "What has happened to your shoes?" "Oh," he said, "I've got those shoes still. I've kept them very carefully." He went into the house and brought out a brown paper parcel and unwrapped the shining shoes. "I keep these for Sunday when I go to church." So we had to teach him about the importance of wearing shoes all the time.

Some years later, at Christmas time, I went again to visit my old mother. Koranaissen came up to visit us. He was riding a horse and was surrounded by a whole group of people whom he had brought from his village—people who had been in his school and their parents and others, all of whom had come to this Christian service that old Granny Brand was holding. ALL of them led by this one-time leprosy beggar, sitting on the horse with quiet dignity and real leadership as an elder of the church.

He was an example of the transforming power of Christ—a man who was found by an old lady who was consumed by the love of Jesus Christ, then went to a place where he was exposed to medical science and all that technology can do, and came back with dignity and manhood and the love of God in him, which he could pass on to other people.

As I came away from the visit to my old mother, I said to her, "Why don't you come home with us this time and have a little rest? Surely, at 85, it is time you had a furlough." She said, "No, the people up here need me, but," she said, "go home and tell them back there about all these mountains, and all these sick people. Tell them about their needs. Tell them that my horse is getting old and that we are both very tired and some other people have got to come out and carry on."

And that is the challenge that I leave with American Leprosy Missions, the challenge of the unreached areas, the challenge of new knowledge, and the challenge that we shall reach out our hands with the Church of God and touch with the Master's touch.

Appendix E

"THE LEPROSY WORKER'S PRAYER"
by Susan S. Renault

Do not dull my pain, Lord.
Do not allow me to see a wounded hand
Instead of a broken heart.
Make my pain acute.
Remind me daily that he is not a patient,
But a father who can no longer farm.
She is not case number 325,
But a mother, outcast and afraid.
Do not dull my fear, Lord,
Lest I forget to feel hers,
This teenager with bent fingers
Hidden in the folds of her sari.
Do not calm my spirit,
Lest I begin to think I am
Just a clerk or just a doctor
Or just a driver or just a nurse.
Give me Your pain,
Your broken heart,
That I might always be
Your compassion,
Your healing touch,
Your love.

Damien and Dutton: Two Josephs on Molokai by Howard E. Crouch. (New York: The Damien-Dutton Society for Leprosy Aid, Inc., 1998).

Doctor Not Afraid by Winifred Kellersberger Vass. (Franklin, Tenn.: Providence House Publishers, 1986).

Don't Treat Me Like I Have Leprosy! by Thomas F. Frist. (London: TALMILEP, 1996).

"The Experience of Self-Care Groups with People Affected by Leprosy: ALERT, Ethiopia" by Catherine Benbow and Teferra Tamiru. *Leprosy Review* (Sept. 2001).

Father Damien: A Journey from Cashmere to His Home in Hawaii by Edward Clifford. (London: MacMillian and Co., 1889).

Fifty Years Work for Lepers: 1874–1924 by unlisted author. (London: The Mission to Lepers, 1924).

Garden in the Wilderness: Mennonite Communities in the Paraguayan Chaco 1927–1997 by Edgar Stoesz and Muriel Stackley. (Winnipeg, Man.: CMBC Publications, 1999).

History of American Leprosy Missions: A Journey of Mercy by Oliver W. Hasselblad, M.D. (N.p., available in ALM Archives).

Hospital Mennonita Km. 81: Liebe, die tatig wird by Gerhard Ratzlaff, Asuncion. (2001) A history on the occasion of the fiftieth anniversary. (Available in German only.)

Our Journey Through Life: The Memoirs of John and Clara Schmidt and Their Family. Available from the Archives of Mennonite Central Committee, Akron, Penn., 17501.

The Lepers of Our Indian Empire: A Visit to Them in 1890–91 by Wellesley C. Bailey. (London: John F. Shaw & Co., 1891).

Mary Reed: Missionary to the Lepers by John Jackson. (London: Marshall Bros., 1899).

"The Mennonite Experience With Leprosy" by Edgar Stoesz. *Mission Focus* 8 (2000).

Ridding the World of Leprosy by William M. Danner and Fleming H. Revell. (New York & Chicago: N.p., 1919).

Thirty-One Banana Leaves by Winifred Kellersberger Vass. (Franklin, Tenn.: Providence House Publishers, 1994).

For a discussion of the similarities and dissimilarities between leprosy and HIV/AIDS, attention is directed to the book, *The Gift Of Pain,* by Paul Brand and Philip Yancey (Grand Rapids, Mich.: Zondervan 1993, 1997). They discuss such topics as the power of stigma, fear of contagion, medical lessons, and the church's response.

International Leprosy Association (ILA), 46, 53, 132, 172, 178
International Leprosy Congress, 46, 53–55, 112, 132, 134, 156, 180, 223
Inthawarorot Suriyawong, Prince of Chiang Mai, 30
Ivory Coast, 136, 183, **181**
Jamkhed (India), 133, 144, 179
Jesudasan, Kumar and Usha, 99
Johnwick, Edgar, 101
Jopling, W. H., 155, 161
José, 107
Kaiser-I-Hind, 21, 125, 218
Karigiri, 98–101, 104, 112, 124, 132, 165, 199, 220, 224
Kellersberger, Edna (née Bosché), 44–45, 47–50
Kellersberger, Eugene, 43–56, 63, 121, 122, 129, 134, 214, 211, **45, 56, 53, 63, 214**
Kellersberger, Julia, 50, 54–56, 214, **56**
Km. 81, 64–70, 73, 126, 131, 173, **65**
Koh Klang Hospital, 29–30, 32, 36, 37
Kongawi, Jacques, **190, 197**
Koop, C. Everett, **110**
Krishnamurthy, John, 86–87, 92
Kumar, 93–94
Kweta, 54
Law, Skinsnes Anwei, 172
Laymen's Missionary Movement, 22
Lehman, Linda, 165, 174, 178, **179**
Leonard Wood Memorial, 46
Leopold, Crown Prince of Belgium (later King), 49–50, 214
Leprosy
  in the Bible, 6
  explained, 8,12
  in USA, 102–3
  major trends in the treatment of, 182
  transmission, 190–91
Leprosy Mission, The (TLMI), 15, 147, 221, 224
Leprosy Plus, 177–86
Leprosy Registry at the Armed Forces Institute of Pathology, 46
"The Leprosy Worker's Prayer," 235
London School of Tropical Medicine, 47
Loong Paeng, 31
Lubilashi, Samuel, **50**
Lusambo, 47
MAP International, 136
Mariam, Senkenesh, 171
Mathew, Thomas, **190**
Maury, Matthew, 169–70
McGilvary, Daniel and Sophia, 27, 29
McKean, James and Laura, 25–40, **29, 34**
McKean Leper Home (later McKean Rehabilitation Center), 25, 35, 37, **37**

Mennonite Central Committee (MCC), 59–60, 64, 70
Meyers, Wayne and Esther, 128
Miller, Orie O., 61, 70, 126, 158
Miracle at Carville, 103
Missena, Nicholas and Antonia, 66–67
Mission to Lepers in India and the Far East, 17
Molokai (Hawaii), 8–11, 13, 120, 219
Muir, Ernest, 53, 55
Multidrug therapy (MDT), 12, 56, 134–35, 157, 161, 177–79, 181, 182–85, 190, 193, 222, **160, 178**
Mycrobacterium leprae (*M. leprae*), 5, 8, 12, 81, 152–57, 160–61, 184, 195–96, **153, 157**
Nai Dobphhromin Chaiworasin, 36, **36**
National Hansen's Disease Museum, 103
New Hearts, New Faces, 122
New York Academy of Science, 122
New York Ecumenical Missionary Conference, 6
Nippon Foundation, 183, 185
Novartis Foundation, 183
On Leprosy, 10
Order of British Empire, 111
Paraguay, 18, 59–74, 131
Penner, Peter and Elizabeth, 21, 62
Pepito, Randy, **190**
Pete the Pig, 38, 128, **38**
Pfaltzgraff, Roy E., 127, 220
Prevention of Disabilities (POD), 167, 172, 178, 182, 185, 195, 224, **179**
Promin, 102, 121, 156, 214
Rambo, Victor, 78–79
Ratzlaff, Gerhard, 67–68, 73
Reed, Mary, 15–16, **16**
Renault, Susan S., 235, **174**
Revell, Fleming H., 17–18, 21–22, 63, **21–22**
Ridding The World of Leprosy, 119
Ridley, Denis, 155, 161
Rifampicin, 191
Rifampin, 102
Rockefeller Foundation, 98, 100
Ross, Emory, 55, 121–22, 213–14, **55, 213**
Ross, Felton, 103, 158, 165, 174, 178, 185, 220, **180**
Ross, Una, **180**
Rozenweig, Helen, 218
Sadan, 85, 88
Saint Francis of Assisi, 9, 142
Sams, John R., 131, 218, 221–22, **110, 222**
Santa Isabel, 64
Sasakawa Memorial Health Foundation, 185
Sasakawa, Yohei, **185**

Saunderson, Paul, **192**
Schieffelin Leprosy Research and Training Centre (*See* Karigiri)
Schieffelin, William Jay, 17–18, 22, 124, **22**
Schmidt, Clara, 59–60, 62, 71, **71**
Schmidt, John, 59–74, 173, **70–71**
Schmidt, Wesley, 73
Scollard, David, **161**
Scott, Waldron, 221, **221**
Scudder, Ida, 77, 123, 213
Sensenig, Dan, 158
Shane, Tim, **190**
Skinner, Julia Lake (*See* Kellersberger, Julia)
Skinsnes, Olaf K., 127, 132, 155, 161
Smith, Cairns, 184
Stigma Elimination Program (STEP), 148
Stroessner, Alfredo, 64
Suggested Readings, 236
Sulfone, 79, 81, 92–93, 102–3, 112, 121, 156
Sunday School Times, 38
Taylor, Clyde, 129
Thailand, 25–40
Thirty-One Banana Leaves, 54
"Touch" (address by Paul Brand), 128, 232–34
Trautman, John, **110**
Tucker, Hugh C., 129
Tulane School of Medicine, 120
Tuttle, Glen W., 130, 218
Tye, Norwood B., 131
U.S. Public Health Service, 101–102, 118, 120, 126, 156
Unruh, Gertrude, 73
Vellore Christian College and Medical Hospital, 77–80, 84–87, 99, 123, 124, 133, 213
Victor Heiser/Heiser Foundation, 132, 155
Vietnam Christian Service, 130
Voth, Nety, 68
Wade, H. W., 46
Watson, Jean, 165, 167, 169, 174
Wiens, Carlos, 69–70
Wilson, Eugene, 218
Without the Camp, 15
Wood, Leonard, 46
Word and Deed Newsletter, 180
World Council of Churches, 129
World Health Organization (WHO), 23, 111, 132, 134, 160, 170, 177, 182, 185, 191, 200, 221–23
World Missionary Conference, 22, 45
Wu, T. C., 120
Yuasa, Yo, 172, 185
Yui Thepniran, 28